Table of Contents

Organic Beauty Products

Recipes

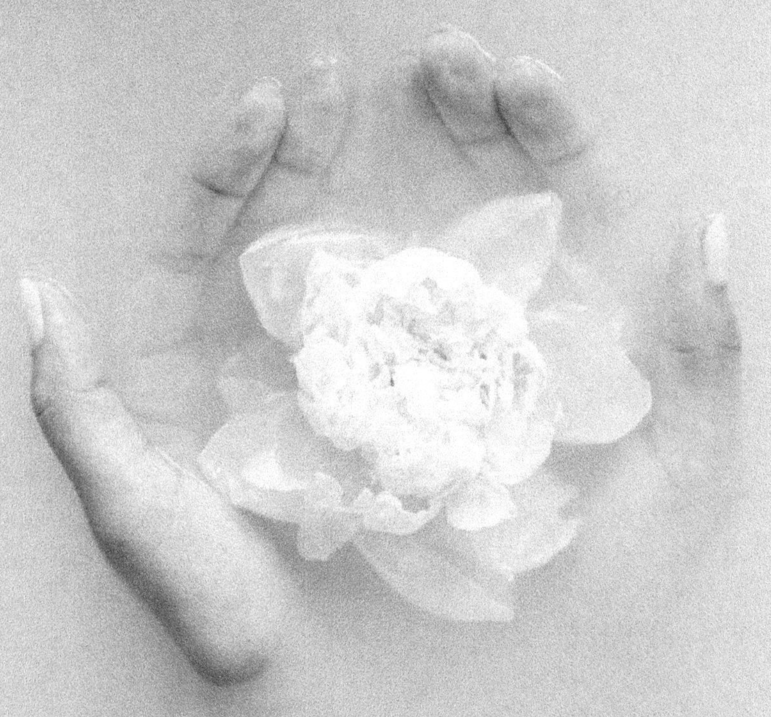

Face Serum Facial Scrub Lipstick Shower Gel & More

Shahaan Merchant

Organic Beauty Products Recipes

By

Shahaan Merchant

All rights reserved. No part of this publication may be reproduced, distributed, or transmitted in any form or by any means, including photocopying, recording, or other electronic or mechanical methods, without the prior written permission of the publisher, except in the case of brief quotations embodied in critical reviews and certain other noncommercial uses permitted by copyright law.

This book is intended for personal use and informational purposes only. The recipes, formulations, methods, and instructions provided herein are the intellectual property of the authors and are protected under copyright law. Any unauthorized reproduction, distribution, or adaptation of the content, in whole or in part, is strictly prohibited and may result in legal action.

Disclaimer

The information provided in this book is for educational and informational purposes only. The recipes, instructions, and formulations shared are based on research and experience but are not guaranteed to be error-free, accurate, or suitable for all individuals or circumstances.While every effort has been made to ensure accuracy, the authors and publishers cannot be held responsible for any adverse reactions, accidents, or damages that may arise from the use, misuse, or application of the information contained herein.

Readers understand and acknowledge that the creation, application, or use of homemade products described in this book carries inherent risks. The authors, publishers, and affiliated parties do not assume any responsibility or liability for the accuracy, completeness, suitability, or outcomes resulting from the utilization of the information presented herein.

Furthermore, the authors and publishers disclaim any responsibility for:

Allergic reactions, skin irritations, or adverse health effects resulting from the use of homemade products, as individual sensitivities vary.

Accidents, damages, or injuries incurred during the production, application, or storage of homemade products.

Any inaccuracies, omissions, or errors in the recipes, formulations, or instructions provided.

Readers are strongly advised to:

Conduct patch tests and seek professional advice before using any homemade products, especially if they have known allergies, sensitivities, or health conditions.

Perform thorough research, including cross-referencing multiple sources, to ensure the safety, suitability, and legality of ingredients and methods used.

Adhere to safety guidelines, including proper storage, handling of ingredients, and compliance with local regulations and laws concerning product manufacturing and distribution.

By using the information in this book, readers agree to hold harmless the authors, publishers, and affiliates from any liability, claims, damages, or expenses that may arise directly or indirectly from the use or misuse of the provided information.

Table of Contents

Turmeric Powder
Rosewater
Baking Soda
Citric Acid
Cornstarch
Epsom Salt
Mica Powder
Granulated Sugar
Vanilla Extract
Brown Sugar
Isopropyl Alcohol (Rubbing Alcohol)
Aloe Vera Gel
Witch Hazel
Vegetable Glycerin
Acetone
Glycerin
Avocado
Cinnamon
Cornstarch
Zinc Oxide Powder
Flaxseeds
Bentonite Clay or Kaolin Clay
Beetroot Powder
Nutmeg
Mica Powder
Activated Charcoal

Organic Recipes Section

Solid Soap Bars
Shampoo
Conditioner Bars
Body Lotion
Lip Balm
Face Mask

Bath Bombs
Body Scrub
Facial Scrub
Massage Oil
Beard Oil
Hand Sanitizer
Bath Salts
Aftershave Lotion
Deodorant
Makeup Remover
Nail Polish Remover
Hand Cream
Hair Mask
Dry Shampoo
Sunscreen
Natural Bug Repellent
Lip Scrub
Makeup Setting Spray
Hair Gel
Hair Serum
Beard Balm
Beard Wash
Cuticle Oil
Bath Oils
Bubble Bath
Shower Gel
Face Toner
Face Serum
Face Cleanser
Eye Cream
Face Moisturizer
Makeup Primer
Makeup Foundation
Blush/Bronzer
Eye Shadow

Mascara
Eyeliner
Lipstick/Lip Gloss
Body Butter
Baby Shampoo/Body Wash
Diaper Rash Cream
Baby Oil
Baby Lotion
Reusable Makeup Remover Pads
Handcrafted Botanical Soaps

Introduction

Ever wondered about the magic behind homemade organic cosmetics? Dive into a world where natural ingredients are the stars!

There are 2 parts in this book. In the first part, explore the essence of various ingredients, their unique traits, and how they contribute to crafting your favorite cosmetics. In the second part there are actual organic cosmetics recipes, which you can start making and treat yourself with the pleasure of going organic and natural. This part unveils the treasure trove of recipes! With detailed instructions and quantities, dive into making your own goodies. Start with these recipes and embark on your journey to becoming a master in crafting natural beauty products.

Empowerment in Creation

With practice and further exploration, you'll not only craft for yourself but could even venture into launching your own line of organic cosmetics! This book is your key to a world where nature's goodness meets beauty.

Embrace the magic of homemade organic cosmetics. Start with understanding the ingredients, move on to creating your favorites, and **who knows, you might just be the next big thing in the world of natural beauty!**

Understanding the nature and properties of ingredients before diving into making products from these recipes is crucial for several reasons:

Safety and Effectiveness

Understanding how each ingredient acts and interacts with others means your homemade products will be safe and effective. Knowing their characteristics prevents dangerous blends or reactions which could make the product worthless or worse, unsafe.

Allergies and Sensitivities

Some people may be allergic or sensitive to particular ingredients. Knowing these things will help you decide what else to use, or do patch tests first to make sure your products are safe for anybody who might use them.

Product Performance

Different ingredients have different effects and roles in a formula. Knowing these properties is important in designing formulations to get what's wanted. For example, learning which oils provide moisture, which act as preservatives, and which give a scent can help you create products that work well.

Sustainability and Eco-friendliness

Knowing about ingredients makes it possible to choose environmentally friendly options. Some could be more sustainable or have a smaller ecological footprint, making them more in line with your ideals and supporting a more eco friendly lifestyle.

Cost-effectiveness

Knowing the properties of ingredients makes it easier to choose wisely and make sound investments, that is to invest in ingredients which can be used in a variety of dishes. This can save money in the long run by cutting down on waste and raising utility levels.

Customization and Innovation

Once you know about properties, you can experiment and come up with your own formulas. Understanding the behavior of each ingredient allows for creative adjustments and substitutions, resulting in unique and personal products.

Legal and Regulatory Compliance

In some areas there may be ingredient restrictions or regulations which you must be aware of. Some ingredients may be subject to legal restrictions, or require special handling, and being aware of these ahead of time avoids complications.

In essence, understanding the type and properties of ingredients is essential to making safe, effective and individualized products. It allows you to make enlightened choices, formulations that are perfect for your needs, and you can have extra peace of mind because the products you produce aren't just practical-they're also safe for you and those around you.

Coconut Oil

This beauty is like a superhero in the world of homemade cosmetics! Extracted from mature coconuts, it's a go-to ingredient for its versatility and nourishing properties. Why do we love it so much? Well, it's a fantastic moisturizer, sinking deep into your skin without feeling greasy. Plus, it's packed with fatty acids that work wonders for softening and smoothing. Coconut oil is a champ in various cosmetics, from lip balms and body lotions to hair masks and makeup removers. It's also a natural antimicrobial, helping to keep skin healthy and protected. Caution-wise, some folks might find it comedogenic, which means it can clog pores for certain skin types. Always give it a test before going all-in!

Olive Oil

The kitchen's golden liquid has a place in skincare too! Olive oil is known for its rich moisturizing abilities and antioxidants. It's gentle and excellent for dry skin, acting as a natural hydrator and softener. You'll find it in body lotions, cleansers, and even as a makeup remover. It's full of goodness like vitamin E and fatty acids, making it a top choice for nourishing your skin. But be mindful—it might feel a bit heavy for some skin types or cause allergic reactions in sensitive folks. Patch test? Always a good idea!

Sweet Almond Oil

This oil's like a magic potion for your skin! Sweet almond oil is light, easily absorbed, and loaded with vitamins E and A. It's super gentle, making it fantastic for sensitive skin. You'll spot it in various cosmetics, from body lotions to facial serums and even as a makeup remover. Sweet almond oil known for its moisturizing and soothing properties, helping to calm irritation and leaving your skin feeling all soft and supple. But, hey, some folks might have nut allergies, so watch out for that and test it out first!

"These oils are like the dream team in homemade cosmetics, each bringing its unique benefits and properties to the table. Always do a little test to make sure your skin loves them as much as we do!"

Jojoba Oil

Let's talk about this golden elixir! Jojoba oil, pronounced "ho-ho-ba," might just become your skin's new BFF. Extracted from the seeds of the jojoba plant, it's a natural marvel. Why is it so special? Well, it's crazy similar to the oils our skin produces naturally, making it a fantastic moisturizer without feeling greasy. This magic oil is a star in cosmetics because it's packed with nutrients like vitamin E, B-complex vitamins, and minerals. It's gentle enough for all skin types, even sensitive ones! Jojoba oil is famous for its hydrating and balancing act on your skin, helping with everything from dryness to oily patches. Oh, and it's a superhero for hair too, bringing shine and softness to those locks. But hey, it's rare, but some folks might have allergic reactions, so patch test before slathering it all over!

Vitamin E Oil

Cue the superhero music! Vitamin E oil like the protector of your skin—it's all about antioxidants and nourishment. Extracted from vitamin E-rich foods or created synthetically, it's a beloved ingredient in cosmetics for its skin-loving properties. Why? Because it's an antioxidant powerhouse, fighting those pesky free radicals that cause skin damage. Vitamin E oil known for its hydrating and healing prowess, helping with scars, dryness, and wrinkles. You'll spot it in face moisturizers, lip balms, and even in sunscreens for that extra shield against UV damage. But watch out—it might cause reactions for some sensitive skin types, so a little patch test can save the day!

Lavender Essential Oil

Ah, the calming scent of lavender! Lavender essential oils like a spa day in a bottle. Extracted from lavender flowers, it's renowned for its soothing and relaxing properties. This oil's a multitasker—it's great for both your skin and mind! Lavender oil's often used in cosmetics for its anti-inflammatory and antiseptic qualities. It's a pro at calming irritated skin and can help with acne or minor burns. Plus, that heavenly scent? It's like an aromatherapy session, calming your nerves and promoting relaxation. It's often added to body lotions, bath bombs, and even face masks for that floral touch. But hey, some folks might be sensitive, so a patch test is always a wise move!

"These oils and essential oils are nature's gift to our homemade cosmetics, bringing their unique benefits to the table. They're like the special ingredients that make our DIY creations even more amazing. Just remember, a little test goes a long way to ensure your skin adores them as much as we do!"

Peppermint Essential Oil

Picture a cool, refreshing breeze on a hot day—that's peppermint essential oil! Extracted from peppermint leaves, it's like a breath of fresh air in the world of cosmetics. Why do we love it? Well, it's a multitasker! Peppermint oil is famous for its invigorating scent and cooling sensation on the skin. It's a champ at relieving sore muscles when added to massage oils and can even help soothe headaches. Plus, it's an antibacterial rockstar, making it a great addition to skincare products like cleansers or toners, helping to keep things clear and fresh. Caution-wise, it's potent stuff! Always dilute it properly, especially for sensitive skin, and avoid using it around delicate areas like the eyes.

Eucalyptus Essential Oil

That clean, crisp scent you associate with spas? That's eucalyptus essential oil! Extracted from eucalyptus leaves, it's a powerhouse of goodness. Why is it such a star in homemade cosmetics? Well, it's a natural decongestant, making it perfect for adding to shower gels or bath bombs for a spa-like experience that can clear your sinuses. It's also antiseptic and can be helpful in treating minor cuts or insect bites. Plus, its refreshing aroma can boost your mood and mental clarity. Caution alert: It's strong! Always dilute it well, especially for sensitive skin, and avoid using it around the eyes.

Argan Oil

Meet the liquid gold of Morocco! Argan oil, derived from the kernels of the argan tree, is like a treasure trove for skin and hair. Why is it so adored? It's a fantastic moisturizer, loaded with antioxidants, fatty acids, and vitamin E. It's super nourishing and can work wonders for dry skin or frizzy hair. In cosmetics, it's often used in body lotions, hair serums, and facial moisturizers for that silky, soft touch. It's lightweight and easily absorbed, making it a hit for all skin types. Caution-wise, while it's great for most, some might find it comedogenic, so give it a test before slathering it all over!

"These essential oils and argan oil bring their unique benefits to our homemade cosmetics, from providing refreshing scents to offering therapeutic properties. Just remember, these oils are powerful, so a little goes a long way! Always patch test and dilute them properly to ensure they work their magic safely and effectively."

Cedarwood Essential Oil

Imagine a stroll through a peaceful forest—that's the essence of cedarwood essential oil! Extracted from the wood of cedar trees, it's like nature's serenity in a bottle. Why do we love it? Well, cedarwood oil is renowned for its grounding, calming properties. It's often used in cosmetics for its soothing effects on the skin and mind. This oil is like a stress-reliever, easing tension and promoting relaxation. It's also great for skincare, as it's a natural antiseptic, helping to combat skin irritations or acne. Caution-wise, it's a potent oil! Always dilute it properly before applying it to the skin, and a little goes a long way in terms of fragrance.

Sandalwood Essential Oil

The sweet, woody aroma of sandalwood essential oil! Derived from the heartwood of sandalwood trees, it's a beloved ingredient in cosmetics for its luxurious scent and therapeutic benefits. Sandalwood oil is like a spa day at home, known for its calming and mood-enhancing properties. It's often used in skincare for its anti-inflammatory and antimicrobial properties, making it excellent for soothing irritated skin or reducing blemishes. Plus, it's great for promoting relaxation and mental clarity. Caution-wise, it's considered safe for most skin types, but as with any essential oil, it's best to do a patch test before full use.

Chamomile Essential Oil

Imagine the gentle touch of a soothing tea—that's chamomile essential oil! Extracted from chamomile flowers, it's a calming powerhouse in the world of cosmetics. Chamomile oil is well-known for its anti-inflammatory and skin-soothing properties. It's like a hug for sensitive or irritated skin, often used in skincare products like serums or moisturizers to calm redness and promote skin healing. Its gentle nature makes it suitable for various skin types, even for little ones, making it a go-to in baby skincare products. Caution-wise, while it's generally safe, some individuals might have allergic reactions, so a patch test is always a smart move.

"These essential oils, like fragrant gems, bring their unique scents and benefits to our homemade cosmetics. They're nature's way of adding a touch of tranquility and care to our skincare routines. Remember, a little goes a long way with essential oils, and diluting them properly ensures they work their magic safely and effectively."

Fractionated Coconut Oil

Coconut's fancy friend! Fractionated coconut oil is like the smooth operator in the world of oils. Unlike regular coconut oil, it stays liquid at room temperature because it's been "fractionated" to remove the long-chain fatty acids. Why do we fancy it? Well, it's lightweight and super absorbent, making it a star moisturizer for your skin without that greasy feeling. It's a gentle giant, suitable for all skin types, and it won't clog those precious pores. Fractionated coconut oil's also fantastic for diluting essential oils or making DIY cosmetics. Caution-wise, it's considered safe for most folks, but always be cautious with allergies, and if you're trying it for the first time, a patch test is a smart move!

Shea Butter

Meet the superhero of hydration! Shea butter's like a nourishing hug for your skin. It's extracted from the nuts of the shea tree and has been used for centuries for its moisturizing and healing properties. Why do we adore it? Well, it's loaded with vitamins A, E, and F, making it a powerhouse for soothing dry, irritated skin. It's a multitasker, helping with everything from reducing inflammation to providing natural UV protection. Shea butter's a go-to in cosmetics for its ability to deeply moisturize without feeling heavy. But hey, some folks might have nut allergies, so patch test before you dive in!

Lye (Sodium Hydroxide)

Here comes the essential ingredient in soap-making! Lye, also known as sodium hydroxide, is like the magician that turns oils into soap. It's a powerful alkali substance that's essential for the saponification process. Why use it? Well, when mixed with fats and oils, it causes a chemical reaction that results in soap. Caution flags high! Lye is caustic and needs to be handled with extreme care—always wear protective gear like gloves and goggles and work in a well-ventilated area. It can cause skin or eye irritation, so be extra cautious. When mixing lye, always add it to water slowly, never the other way around. Safety first, always!

"These ingredients, like the stars of our DIY cosmetic show, bring their unique properties and benefits to our homemade creations. They're the magic ingredients that make our products so wonderful, but always remember to handle them with care and caution for safe and effective use."

Liquid Castile Soap

Imagine a gentle, multi-talented soap—welcome to liquid castile soap! Made from plant oils, it's a star in natural skincare. Why do we adore it? Well, it's a mild cleanser suitable for various skin types, even sensitive ones. Liquid castile soap doesn't contain harsh chemicals or synthetic detergents, making it a go-to for folks aiming for a natural skincare routine. It's versatile too! You can use it as a base for homemade shampoos, body washes, or even as a household cleaner. But remember, it's concentrated, so a little goes a long way. Caution-wise, while it's generally safe, some might find it drying due to its cleansing properties, so follow up with a moisturizer.

Coconut Milk

The creamy goodness of coconut milk! Extracted from grated coconut flesh, it's not just for cooking—it's a skincare delight too. Why do we love it? It's packed with nutrients like vitamins C, E, B1, B3, B5, and B6, making it a hydrating powerhouse. Coconut milk's excellent at moisturizing dry skin and soothing irritation. It's often used in cosmetics for its nourishing properties in body lotions, hair masks, or even as a base for facial cleansers. Caution-wise, while it's a fantastic natural moisturizer, some individuals might be sensitive or allergic, so a patch test is wise, especially if it's your first time using it.

Cocoa Butter

Meet the delicious-smelling, ultra-nourishing cocoa butter! Extracted from cocoa beans, it's like a dessert for your skin. Why do we adore it? It's incredibly rich in fatty acids and antioxidants, perfect for hydrating and protecting the skin. Cocoa butter's a champ at softening dry or chapped skin, and its emollient properties make it a popular ingredient in lip balms, body butters, and lotions. It's even said to help fade scars and stretch marks! Caution-wise, while it's generally safe, some might find it comedogenic, so test it on a small area before widespread use.

"These ingredients bring their unique benefits to our homemade cosmetics, providing natural goodness to keep our skin happy and healthy. Just remember, each skin is unique, so patch test and find what works best for you!"

Beeswax

Picture the honeycombs made by bees—that's beeswax! It's a waxy substance secreted by honeybees, and it's a superhero in homemade cosmetics. Why do we love it? Well, it's a natural thickener and emulsifier, adding that creamy texture to lotions and balms without feeling greasy. Beeswax creates a protective barrier on the skin, sealing in moisture without clogging pores. Plus, it's a rockstar in lip balms, giving them that perfect consistency and locking in moisture to keep those lips oh-so-kissable. Caution-wise, it's generally safe, but some people might be allergic to bee products, so a patch test is wise.

Apple Cider Vinegar

It's not just for salads—it's a game-changer in cosmetics too! Apple cider vinegar is made by fermenting crushed apples and it's a natural wonder for your skin and hair. Why do we swear by it? It's like a balancing act for your skin's pH levels, keeping things in check and helping to fight acne or soothe irritated skin. For hair, it can act as a clarifying rinse, removing buildup and giving your locks that extra shine. But hold your horses, it's potent stuff! Always dilute it before use, especially on sensitive skin or scalp, and avoid your eyes.

Arrowroot Powder

Meet the unsung hero in cosmetics! Arrowroot powder is a silky-smooth powder derived from the rhizomes of tropical plants. Why is it a star? Well, it's a natural alternative to talc or cornstarch, often used in skincare products to absorb moisture without clogging pores. It's a soft touch, perfect for homemade deodorants, body powders, or even as a thickener in lotions. Plus, it's gentle on sensitive skin and can soothe irritation. Caution-wise, it's generally safe, but always do a patch test to be sure, especially if you have sensitive skin.

"These ingredients bring their unique benefits to our homemade cosmetics, from providing texture and thickness to adding that special touch of natural care. But remember, every skin reacts differently, so patch testing is your trusty pal to ensure these ingredients work their magic safely and effectively for you!"

Oatmeal

The unsung hero in our morning bowls and skincare routines! Oatmeal isn't just for breakfast—it's a soothing, skin-loving wonder. Why do we adore it? Well, it's loaded with goodness like antioxidants and anti-inflammatory properties, making it a gentle exfoliator that helps soothe irritated skin. In homemade cosmetics, it's like a magician that calms sensitive skin, unclogs pores, and helps with pesky skin conditions like eczema or acne. Plus, it's an excellent addition to scrubs and masks, gently buffing away dead skin cells to reveal that fresh glow. Caution-wise, it's usually safe for most skin types, but those with oat allergies might need to be cautious.

Honey

That sweet, golden goodness isn't just for sweetening tea—it's a skincare superstar too! Honey, particularly raw honey, is like a treasure trove of skin-loving properties. Why do we swear by it? Well, it's antibacterial, helping fight acne-causing bacteria, and it's super moisturizing too. Honey's antioxidants can help slow down aging, leaving your skin looking radiant and youthful. In DIY cosmetics, it's often used in masks, cleansers, or even as a spot treatment. Caution-wise, while it's generally safe, it might cause irritation for some sensitive skin types or those allergic to bee products, so a patch test is a good idea.

Plain Yogurt

Move over, breakfast bowl—yogurt's also a star in skincare! Plain yogurt isn't just delicious; it's packed with goodies like lactic acid, a gentle exfoliator that helps brighten skin and reduce discoloration. It's like a natural moisturizer too, leaving skin feeling soft and supple. In homemade cosmetics, it's often used in masks or cleansers for its soothing and hydrating properties. Plus, it contains probiotics that can help maintain healthy skin flora. Caution-wise, it's generally safe, but those with dairy allergies might want to skip this ingredient.

"These kitchen staples aren't just for your morning routine—they're fantastic ingredients in our homemade cosmetics, adding their natural goodness to keep our skin happy, healthy, and glowing. Always remember, patch testing is the secret sauce to ensure these ingredients work their magic safely for you!"

Turmeric Powder

Turmeric, that golden spice found in your pantry, isn't just for cooking—it's a skincare gem too! Why is it so cool? Well, turmeric is packed with antioxidants and has anti-inflammatory properties that can be a boon for your skin. It's been used for centuries to help with acne, blemishes, and even out skin tone. When used in homemade cosmetics, like masks or scrubs, it can work wonders, leaving your skin looking brighter and feeling refreshed. But, a word of caution—it's vibrant and can stain, so be careful with clothing and surfaces. Also, some might be sensitive to it, so a patch test is a good idea before going all-in.

Rosewater

The sweet scent of roses—rosewater isn't just a pretty fragrance, it's a skincare multitasker! Made from the petals of roses, it's like a gentle hug for your skin. Why do we adore it? It's a natural astringent, helping to balance skin pH, reduce redness, and soothe irritation. Plus, it's hydrating and refreshing, making it a go-to in toners or facial mists. In homemade cosmetics, it's often used for its calming and anti-inflammatory properties. Caution-wise, it's generally safe, but as with anything new, it's good to do a patch test to be sure.

Baking Soda

From baking bread to beautifying your skin, baking soda wears many hats! It's a household staple with exfoliating properties that can help slough off dead skin cells, leaving your skin feeling smooth and looking fresh. When used in homemade cosmetics, like gentle scrubs, it can help unclog pores and balance oiliness. However, it's powerful stuff, so it's crucial to use it sparingly and with caution. Overuse might cause dryness or irritation, especially for those with sensitive skin. A patch test is always a smart move!

"These everyday ingredients aren't just for the kitchen—they're versatile additions to our skincare routines. They bring their own unique benefits, but as with any new skincare product, it's wise to test them out gently to ensure they suit your skin just right!"

Citric Acid

Citric acid isn't just that tangy stuff in citrus fruits—it's a versatile helper in homemade cosmetics! Wondering why it's cool? Well, it's a natural preservative, helping our skincare creations last longer without the need for harsh chemicals. Plus, it's an ace at balancing pH levels, which is great for maintaining healthy skin. In bath bombs and some cleansers, it adds that fizz and effervescence we love! However, a gentle heads-up: It's potent, so using too much might cause irritation, especially for sensitive skin. A little goes a long way!

Cornstarch

Cornstarch, a pantry staple, isn't just for thickening sauces—it's a gentle powerhouse in homemade cosmetics! It's prized for its ability to absorb excess oil and moisture, making it perfect for body powders or dry shampoos. Its silky texture feels fantastic on the skin, leaving it feeling smooth and velvety. When used appropriately, it can also be calming for irritated skin. But remember, too much can lead to a chalky feel, so balance is key!

Epsom Salt

Ah, Epsom salt—the unsung hero of relaxation! It's not your regular table salt; it's packed with magnesium sulfate, which can work wonders for tired muscles and overall relaxation. In homemade bath salts, it's a gem, helping to soothe aches, pains, and even stress. Plus, it can exfoliate gently, leaving your skin feeling silky soft. Yet, here's a little caution: Using too much can leave your skin feeling dry, so moderate amounts are best.

"These everyday ingredients aren't just kitchen essentials—they're fantastic additions to our homemade cosmetics, offering their unique benefits to keep our skin feeling happy and looking fabulous! Remember, balance and moderation are key when playing with these wonderful ingredients!"

Mica Powder

Imagine a sprinkle of stardust in your cosmetics—that's the charm of mica powder! It's a mineral-based shimmer that adds that dazzling, sparkly effect to your makeup. From eye shadows to blushes and lipsticks, it's the secret ingredient that brings that glamorous glow. But, a gentle caution: Ensure it's cosmetic-grade, as industrial versions might not be safe for skin use. A little tip: A little goes a long way, so sprinkle with caution for that radiant shine!

Granulated Sugar

Sweetness isn't just for cookies; it's a secret beauty ingredient too! Granulated sugar isn't just delightful in baked goods; it's a star in exfoliating scrubs. Those granules work like tiny magic wands, buffing away dead skin cells, leaving your skin super smooth and refreshed. Yet, be gentle! It can be a tad abrasive, so for delicate facial skin, a softer touch might be best. But for rougher areas like elbows or feet, it's perfect to banish dryness!

Vanilla Extract

The sweet aroma of vanilla— it's not just for baking wonders! In cosmetics, it brings a delightful scent that's both comforting and enticing. Think of it as a fragrant hug for your homemade creations! It's often used in lip balms, lotions, or even hair products for that divine aroma. Yet, a small tip: Always opt for pure vanilla extract and not artificial versions, especially for skincare—it's like choosing fresh ingredients for your favorite recipe!

"These everyday items aren't just kitchen essentials; they're secret weapons in the world of homemade cosmetics, adding sparkle, sweetness, and fragrance to our delightful creations! Remember, a touch of these can make your homemade products simply marvelous!"

Brown Sugar

Brown sugar isn't just for sweetening desserts; it's a sweet treat for your skin too! Its fine texture makes it a gentle exfoliant, perfect for scrubs. The grains delicately slough away dead skin cells, leaving your skin softer and smoother, with a natural glow. A tip: Its softer texture makes it ideal for sensitive areas like the face, but it's a bit too harsh for sensitive facial skin, so a lighter touch might be best. For tougher spots like elbows or feet, it works wonders to banish dryness, giving you that silky feel.

Isopropyl Alcohol (Rubbing Alcohol)

This might seem more like a first-aid kit staple, but in cosmetics, it serves as a germ buster! It's often used as a disinfectant in homemade products like hand sanitizers and facial toners. However, a word of caution: It's powerful stuff, so use it wisely and carefully, especially on the skin. Dilution is key! Mixing it with other soothing ingredients is a good idea to keep it gentle yet effective.

Aloe Vera Gel

This ingredient is like a green superhero for the skin! It's known for its cooling, soothing properties, making it a go-to for treating sunburns or calming irritated skin. Beyond its healing powers, it's a hydrating champion too. When used in lotions or gels, it helps lock in moisture, leaving your skin feeling refreshed. But keep an eye out for pure aloe vera gel without added chemicals. It's the natural goodness that makes it a star player in your homemade skincare lineup!

Witch Hazel

Witch hazel might sound like a mystical potion, but it's actually a natural astringent derived from the witch hazel shrub. Its superpower lies in its ability to gently cleanse and tone the skin. It's often used in skincare due to its anti-inflammatory and antioxidant properties. This makes it fantastic for reducing redness, calming irritated skin, and even helping with conditions like acne or eczema. Plus, it's gentle, making it suitable for sensitive skin types. A little goes a long way! But keep an eye out for alcohol-free versions, as alcohol can dry out the skin.

Vegetable Glycerin

Here's a skincare hero that loves to lock in moisture! Vegetable glycerin is a clear, odorless liquid derived from vegetable oils. Its magical touch lies in its humectant properties, which means it attracts moisture from the air into your skin. This makes it an excellent ingredient for hydrating products like lotions, creams, and soaps. It not only moisturizes but also helps maintain the skin's natural barrier, leaving it soft and supple. However, it's wise to dilute it as using it directly might draw moisture out of your skin if the air is dry.

Acetone

Acetone is a powerful solvent often used in nail polish removers. Its main job is to break down and dissolve nail polish quickly and efficiently. While effective, it's important to use acetone with caution. It's a potent chemical that can strip moisture from the nails and surrounding skin, leaving them dry and brittle. If using acetone-based products, remember to moisturize your nails and cuticles afterward to counter its drying effects. Additionally, try not to use acetone too frequently as it can weaken the nails over time. Consider using acetone-free alternatives for gentler nail care.

Glycerin

Glycerin, a clear, odorless liquid, is a true superstar in the world of skincare. It's a natural humectant, which is a fancy way of saying it draws moisture from the air into your skin, keeping it hydrated and supple. This magic ingredient not only moisturizes but also helps to maintain the skin's protective barrier, preventing dryness and roughness. You'll often find it in various skincare products like lotions, soaps, and creams. It's gentle on the skin and suits most skin types, even sensitive ones. But remember, a little goes a long way! Too much glycerin might make the skin feel sticky. Also, look out for glycerin derived from plant sources for the most natural and skin-loving benefits.

Avocado

Avocado isn't just for guacamole; it's a nourishing treat for your skin! Packed with healthy fats, vitamins, and antioxidants, avocado is a boon for dry or damaged skin. Its natural oils deeply moisturize and soften the skin, leaving it feeling smooth and rejuvenated. Avocado is often used in skincare recipes like masks, creams, or oils due to its ability to hydrate and soothe. The vitamins E and C in avocados help in maintaining skin health by protecting it from free radicals and promoting collagen production. However, some people might be allergic to avocado, so it's essential to do a patch test before applying it widely on the skin.

Cinnamon

Beyond its delightful aroma in baking, cinnamon also offers some benefits for skin health. Its antibacterial and antifungal properties can help fight acne-causing bacteria and fungi, making it a potential ingredient in acne-fighting face masks or scrubs. It also has antioxidants that might help in reducing skin inflammation and irritation. However, cinnamon can be potent and might cause skin irritation or allergic reactions, especially when used in high concentrations or on sensitive skin. It's advisable to dilute it properly and conduct a patch test before applying it widely to ensure your skin agrees with it.

Cornstarch

Cornstarch, derived from corn kernels, isn't just for thickening sauces in the kitchen—it has fantastic properties for skincare and cosmetics too! This fine powder is incredibly absorbent, making it an excellent ingredient in homemade cosmetics. It's often used in body powders, bath bombs, and dry shampoos to help absorb excess moisture and oil, leaving your skin feeling dry and silky. Additionally, cornstarch has a soothing effect on irritated or itchy skin, making it a great addition to creams or lotions for calming irritated areas. However, some people might be sensitive or allergic to cornstarch, so a patch test is advisable before using it extensively on the skin.

Zinc Oxide Powder

Zinc oxide might remind you of the white paste your mom used to apply for sun protection, and rightly so! It's a natural mineral that provides powerful protection against the sun's harmful UV rays. This ingredient is the superhero in natural sunscreen formulations due to its ability to create a barrier that reflects and scatters UV radiation. Apart from its sun-blocking prowess, zinc oxide also has skin-calming properties, making it ideal for soothing irritated or sensitive skin. It's non-comedogenic, meaning it won't clog pores, making it suitable for various skincare products like creams and lotions. Yet, some people might experience allergic reactions, so a patch test is recommended, especially for those with sensitive skin.

Flaxseeds

Flaxseeds aren't just a superfood for your diet; they offer impressive benefits for your skin and hair too! The seeds are rich in omega-3 fatty acids, antioxidants, and vitamins, making them a fantastic addition to homemade cosmetics. When ground into a fine powder or used as an oil infusion, flaxseeds become a nourishing treat for the skin and hair. In skincare, they can offer hydration, reduce inflammation, and soothe irritation, making them a valuable ingredient in masks, scrubs, or moisturizers. For hair care, flaxseed gel or oil can add moisture, shine, and strength to your locks. However, individuals allergic to flaxseeds should avoid using them in cosmetics, and a patch test is advisable for first-time use to ensure compatibility with your skin.

Bentonite Clay or Kaolin Clay

Clays like bentonite or kaolin are go-to ingredients in natural skincare routines. These clays boast amazing detoxifying properties, making them stars in face masks and body scrubs. Bentonite clay, sourced from volcanic ash, has strong absorptive qualities, drawing out impurities and excess oil from the skin. It's fantastic for acne-prone or oily skin types. On the other hand, kaolin clay, known for its gentle nature, suits sensitive skin and works wonders in providing a deep yet gentle cleanse. Caution-wise, it's essential to mix these clays with non-reactive substances like water or carrier oils and avoid using metal utensils as they can reduce their effectiveness.

Beetroot Powder

Beetroot powder, derived from dried beets, brings a natural pop of color to cosmetics. It's a vibrant, earthy-colored pigment used to add hues to lip balms, blushes, and even tinted lip glosses. Besides its stunning color, beetroot powder contains antioxidants and vitamins that offer a boost of nourishment for your skin. Caution is necessary when adding beetroot powder to formulations as it may stain fabric and may require preservatives to prevent bacterial growth.

Nutmeg

This aromatic spice isn't just for baking; it's a skincare secret too! Nutmeg, when finely ground, becomes a gentle exfoliant, making it perfect for facial scrubs. Its antibacterial properties can help combat acne and soothe inflammation. However, nutmeg can be potent, so it's essential to use it sparingly and perform a patch test to avoid skin irritation.

Mica Powder

Mica powder is the magical ingredient behind shimmer and sparkle in cosmetics like eyeshadows, highlighters, and body glitter. It offers a reflective sheen and comes in various colors, adding that dazzling effect to makeup. Caution-wise, opt for cosmetic-grade mica to ensure safety and avoid using it near the eyes in loose form.

Activated Charcoal

Activated charcoal, a potent absorber of impurities and toxins, is a superhero ingredient in skincare. It's excellent for drawing out dirt and excess oil, making it a staple in face masks, cleansers, and acne treatments. It can be drying, so it's essential to balance it with hydrating ingredients and use it intermittently.

"Each of these ingredients brings unique benefits to homemade cosmetics, adding color, texture, and skincare benefits. Just remember, a little goes a long way, and it's crucial to patch-test new ingredients to ensure they suit your skin!"

Ingredients:

- Coconut Oil - 400 grams
- Olive Oil - 200 grams
- Shea Butter - 150 grams
- Lye (Sodium Hydroxide) - 138 grams
- Water - 320 grams
- Essential Oils (optional for fragrance) - 30-40 drops

Equipment/Tools:

- Safety goggles and gloves
- Digital kitchen scale
- Stainless steel or heat-resistant plastic mixing bowls
- Silicone or heat-resistant plastic spatulas
- Soap mold(s) (silicone molds work well)
- Immersion blender or hand whisk
- Thermometer
- Protective clothing (long sleeves, apron)

Safety Precautions:

- Always wear safety goggles and gloves when handling lye.
- Work in a well-ventilated area.
- Ensure pets and children are not present during the soap-making process.

Method:

Prepare Your Workspace:

- Lay down newspaper or protective covering on your workspace.
- Set up your equipment and tools.

Safety Gear:

- Put on your safety goggles, gloves, and protective clothing.

Prepare Lye Solution:

- Carefully measure the required amount of water in a heat-resistant container.

- In a separate container, measure the lye crystals.

- CAUTION: Always add lye to water, never water to lye. Slowly add the lye to the water while stirring continuously. This mixture will heat up and release fumes, so do this step in a well-ventilated area. Allow the lye solution to cool down to around 100°F (38°C).

Melt Oils and Butters:

- In a separate heat-resistant bowl, combine the coconut oil, olive oil, and shea butter.

- Gently heat this mixture until all the oils and butter have melted. Aim for a temperature around 100-110°F (38-43°C).

Prepare Soap Base:

- Once both the lye solution and oil mixture are around 100°F (38°C), carefully pour the lye solution into the oils.

- Use an immersion blender or hand whisk to blend the mixture until it reaches trace. Trace is when the mixture thickens to a pudding-like consistency and a trail or "trace" of the mixture remains on the surface before sinking back in.

- Add essential oils at trace and mix thoroughly.

Pour into Molds:

- Pour the soap mixture into the soap molds. Tap the molds gently on the counter to release any air bubbles.

- Cover the molds with a sheet of wax paper and then a towel or blanket to insulate.

Curing Process:

- Let the soap sit in the molds for 24-48 hours.

- After this initial period, remove the soap from the molds and cut it into bars if needed.

- Place the bars on a rack in a well-ventilated area to cure for 4-6 weeks. This allows excess moisture to evaporate, resulting in harder, longer-lasting bars.

Label and Store:

- Once cured, label your soap bars with the date and type of soap.
- Store the bars in a cool, dry place away from direct sunlight.

Notes:

- Remember, accuracy in measuring ingredients, especially lye, is crucial for the success and safety of soap making.
- Always run your recipe through a lye calculator to ensure accuracy in measurements and to determine the correct amount of lye needed for the specific oils and quantities used.

Ingredients:

- Liquid Castile Soap - 1/2 cup
- Coconut Milk - 1/4 cup
- Sweet Almond Oil - 1/2 teaspoon
- Essential Oils (optional for fragrance) - 10-15 drops (lavender, rosemary, tea tree, etc.)
- Distilled Water - 3/4 cup

Equipment/Tools:

- Mixing bowl
- Whisk or spoon for stirring
- Funnel
- Pump dispenser bottle(s)

Method:

Prepare Your Workspace:

Ensure your workspace is clean and sanitized. Sterilize the pump dispenser bottle(s) by washing them thoroughly with hot, soapy water and allowing them to dry completely.

Mix the Ingredients:

- In a mixing bowl, pour the liquid castile soap.

- Add the coconut milk, sweet almond oil, and essential oils (if using).

- Gradually add the distilled water while stirring continuously to avoid excessive foaming.

Stir Well:

Use a whisk or spoon to thoroughly mix all the ingredients. Stir until the mixture is well combined.

Transfer to Dispenser Bottle:

- Use a funnel to pour the prepared shampoo mixture into the clean, dry pump dispenser bottle(s).

- Leave a little space at the top of the bottle to allow for the pump mechanism.

Label and Store:

Label the bottle with the date and type of shampoo. Store it in a cool, dry place away from direct sunlight.

Additional Tips:

- Customization: Experiment with different essential oils to create a fragrance that suits your preferences.
- Shake Before Use: Shake the bottle gently before each use to ensure the ingredients are well mixed.
- Adjust Consistency: If you prefer a thicker shampoo, reduce the amount of water slightly. For a thinner consistency, add a bit more water.

This homemade shampoo is free from harsh chemicals and can be a gentle and nourishing alternative for your hair.

Ingredients:

- Shea Butter - 1/4 cup
- Cocoa Butter - 1/4 cup
- Coconut Oil - 1/4 cup
- Jojoba Oil - 1 tablespoon
- Beeswax - 2 tablespoons
- Apple Cider Vinegar - 2 tablespoons
- Essential Oils (optional for fragrance) - 10-15 drops (lavender, rosemary, etc.)

Equipment/Tools:

- Double boiler or microwave-safe bowl
- Mixing bowl
- Silicon molds or ice cube trays
- Whisk or spoon for stirring

Method:

Prepare Your Workspace:

- Lay out all your ingredients and tools in a clean and sanitized workspace.

Melt Solid Ingredients:

- In a double boiler or microwave-safe bowl, melt the shea butter, cocoa butter, coconut oil, and beeswax together. If using a microwave, use short intervals and stir frequently to avoid overheating.

Combine Oils:

- Once melted and well combined, remove the mixture from heat.

- Add the jojoba oil and essential oils (if using). Stir well to ensure even distribution.

Add Apple Cider Vinegar:

- Slowly add the apple cider vinegar to the mixture while stirring continuously. Be careful as the mixture might fizz a little due to the reaction with the vinegar.

Pour into Molds:

- Pour the conditioner mixture into silicone molds or ice cube trays. Tap the molds gently on the counter to release any air bubbles.

Allow to Set:

- Let the conditioner bars cool and solidify at room temperature for several hours or until completely hardened.

Remove from Molds:

- Once hardened, carefully remove the conditioner bars from the molds. If using larger molds, you can cut the bars into smaller sizes for ease of use.

Storage:

- Store the conditioner bars in a cool, dry place away from direct sunlight. You can wrap them individually in wax paper or store them in airtight containers.

Additional Tips:

- Customization: Feel free to adjust the quantity of essential oils for your preferred fragrance strength.
- Usage: To use, rub the conditioner bar between your hands or directly onto wet hair after shampooing. Massage the conditioner into your hair and rinse thoroughly.

These conditioner bars are free from harsh chemicals and can provide nourishment and conditioning to your hair in a convenient solid form.

Ingredients:

- Shea Butter - 1/4 cup
  - Cocoa Butter - 1/4 cup
- Coconut Oil - 1/4 cup
- Sweet Almond Oil - 2 tablespoons
- Jojoba Oil - 2 tablespoons
- Vitamin E Oil - 1 teaspoon
- Arrowroot Powder - 1 teaspoon (optional for a less greasy feel)
- Essential Oils (optional for fragrance) - 20-30 drops (lavender, chamomile, etc.)

Equipment/Tools:

- Double boiler or microwave-safe bowl
  - Mixing bowl
- Hand mixer or whisk
- Clean and dry jars or containers for storage

Method:

Prepare Your Workspace:

- Ensure your workspace is clean and sanitized. Have all your ingredients and tools ready.

Melt Solid Ingredients:

- In a double boiler or microwave-safe bowl, melt the shea butter, cocoa butter, and coconut oil together. Stir occasionally until fully melted and combined.

Add Liquid Oils:

- Remove the mixture from heat and allow it to cool slightly.

- Add the sweet almond oil, jojoba oil, and vitamin E oil. Stir well to combine.

Optional: Add Arrowroot Powder:

- If you prefer a less greasy feel, you can add arrowroot powder to the mixture and stir until smooth.

Cool the Mixture:

- Allow the mixture to cool to room temperature. You can speed up the process by placing it in the refrigerator for a short while, but don't let it solidify completely.

Whip the Lotion:

- Using a hand mixer or whisk, whip the mixture until it becomes creamy and light in texture. This may take several minutes, so be patient.

Add Essential Oils:

- Once the lotion reaches the desired consistency, add the essential oils for fragrance. Mix well to distribute the scent evenly.

Transfer to Containers:

- Spoon the whipped body lotion into clean and dry jars or containers for storage. Ensure the containers are airtight to preserve the lotion.

Label and Store:

- Label the containers with the date and type of lotion.
- Store the lotion in a cool, dry place away from direct sunlight.

Additional Tips:

● Usage: Apply the homemade body lotion to clean skin as needed, gently massaging it in until absorbed.

● Customization: Experiment with different essential oil blends to create your preferred scent profile.

● Consistency: If the lotion is too thick, you can remelt it and add a bit more liquid oil. If it's too thin, you can refrigerate it to firm up slightly.

This homemade body lotion is rich in natural oils and can help moisturize and nourish your skin without the use of harsh chemicals.

Ingredients:

- Beeswax - 1 tablespoon
- Shea Butter - 1 tablespoon
- Coconut Oil - 1 tablespoon
- Sweet Almond Oil - 1 tablespoon
- Vitamin E Oil - 1/2 teaspoon (optional, for added nourishment)
- Essential Oils (optional for fragrance) - 10-15 drops (peppermint, lavender, etc.)

Equipment/Tools:

- Double boiler or microwave-safe bowl
- Small heat-resistant containers or lip balm tubes
- Dropper or small funnel
- Mixing spoon or spatula

Method:

Prepare Your Workspace:

- Ensure your workspace is clean and sanitized. Gather all your ingredients and tools.

Melt Solid Ingredients:

- In a double boiler or microwave-safe bowl, melt the beeswax, shea butter, and coconut oil together. If using a microwave, use short intervals and stir frequently to avoid overheating.

Add Liquid Oils:

- Once melted and well combined, remove the mixture from heat.

• Add the sweet almond oil and vitamin E oil (if using). Stir well to combine.

Optional: Add Essential Oils:

• If you'd like to add fragrance, add the essential oils drop by drop and mix thoroughly. Essential oils can be potent, so start with a small amount and adjust to your preference.

Pour into Containers:

• Carefully pour the melted lip balm mixture into small heat-resistant containers or lip balm tubes using a dropper or small funnel. Fill them almost to the top, leaving a little space for settling.

Allow to Set:

• Let the lip balm cool and solidify at room temperature for several hours or until completely hardened.

Cap and Store:

• Once hardened, cap the containers securely. Store them in a cool, dry place away from direct sunlight.

Additional Tips:

• Variations: You can customize your lip balm by adding natural colorants like beetroot powder or cocoa powder for tinted balms.

• Usage: Apply the homemade lip balm to your lips as needed to keep them moisturized and protected.

• Gift Idea: These homemade lip balms make fantastic gifts when presented in decorative containers or tubes.

This DIY lip balm is a nourishing and protective solution for dry or chapped lips, made with natural ingredients to keep your lips soft and hydrated.

Ingredients:

- Oatmeal - 2 tablespoons (ground into a fine powder)
- Honey - 1 tablespoon
- Plain Yogurt - 1 tablespoon
- Turmeric Powder - 1/2 teaspoon (optional, for its anti-inflammatory properties)
- Rosewater - 1 teaspoon (optional, for a refreshing scent)

Equipment/Tools:

- Mixing bowl
- Spoon or spatula for mixing
- Small container for storage (if preparing extra)

Method:

Prepare Your Workspace:

- Ensure your workspace is clean and sanitized. Gather all the necessary ingredients and tools.

Prepare Oatmeal:

- Grind the oatmeal in a food processor or blender until it becomes a fine powder. This helps create a smoother consistency for the mask.

Mix Ingredients:

- In a mixing bowl, combine the ground oatmeal, honey, plain yogurt, turmeric powder (if using), and rosewater (if using). Stir the ingredients together until well blended.

Adjust Consistency (Optional):

- If the mixture is too thick, add a bit more yogurt or rosewater to achieve a spreadable consistency. If it's too runny, add a bit more oatmeal.

Apply the Mask:

- Before applying the mask, cleanse your face to remove any makeup or dirt.

- Using clean fingers or a brush, apply an even layer of the mask to your face, avoiding the eye area.

Relax and Let It Dry:

- Allow the mask to dry on your face for about 15-20 minutes. You may feel a tightening sensation as the mask dries.

Rinse Off:

- Once the mask is dry, dampen your face with warm water and gently massage in circular motions to exfoliate before rinsing off the mask completely.

Moisturize:

- Pat your face dry with a clean towel and follow up with your favorite moisturizer to lock in hydration.

Additional Tips:

- Patch Test: Before using the mask on your face, perform a patch test on a small area of skin to ensure you don't have any adverse reactions.
- Frequency: You can use this mask once or twice a week as part of your skincare routine.

This homemade face mask is designed to help exfoliate, nourish, and brighten your skin using natural ingredients known for their skincare benefits. Adjust the ingredients according to your skin's sensitivity and needs.

Ingredients:

- Baking Soda - 1 cup
    - Citric Acid - 1/2 cup
- Cornstarch - 1/2 cup
- Epsom Salt - 1/2 cup
- Coconut Oil - 2 tablespoons (melted)
- Water - 1-2 teaspoons
- Essential Oils - 20-30 drops (lavender, eucalyptus, etc.)
- Natural Food Coloring or Mica Powder (optional for color)

Equipment/Tools:

- Mixing bowls
    - Whisk
- Bath bomb molds (or muffin tin, silicone molds, or even hands for shaping)
- Spray bottle (filled with water)
- Airtight container for storage

Method:

Prepare Your Workspace:

- Ensure your workspace is clean and dry. Gather all the ingredients and tools needed.

Mix Dry Ingredients:

- In a mixing bowl, combine the baking soda, citric acid, cornstarch, and Epsom salt. Use a whisk to break up any clumps and ensure even mixing.

Mix Wet Ingredients:

- In a separate small bowl, mix the melted coconut oil, essential oils, and natural food coloring or mica powder (if using). Mix well to distribute the color evenly.

Combine Wet and Dry Ingredients:

- Slowly add the wet ingredients mixture to the dry ingredients while whisking continuously. Make sure to incorporate the wet ingredients thoroughly into the dry mixture. The mixture should hold together when squeezed without being too wet.

Spritz with Water:

- Using a spray bottle, lightly spritz the mixture with water while continuously mixing with your hands or the whisk. Add water a little at a time until the mixture sticks together when pressed without crumbling.

Pack into Molds:

- Fill each half of your bath bomb molds with the mixture, packing it in tightly. If you're using other molds or shaping by hand, firmly press the mixture into the desired shape.

Press and Release:

- Gently press the mixture into the molds and then carefully release the bath bombs onto a tray or parchment paper. Allow them to dry and harden for at least 24 hours in a dry place.

Store and Enjoy:

- Once completely dry and hardened, store the bath bombs in an airtight container until you're ready to use them.

Additional Tips:

● Experiment with Shapes: Get creative with different molds or shapes for your bath bombs, but ensure they're firm enough to hold the mixture.

● Fragrance and Color: Customize your bath bombs with different essential oils and colors to create a variety of scents and hues.

These homemade bath bombs can add a luxurious touch to your bath experience and can make lovely gifts when packaged beautifully. Adjust the ingredients and scents to suit your preferences.

Ingredients:

- Granulated Sugar - 1 cup
  - Coconut Oil - 1/4 cup (melted but not hot)
- Essential Oils - 10-15 drops (lavender, lemon, peppermint, etc.)
- Vanilla Extract - 1 teaspoon (optional for fragrance)

Equipment/Tools:

- Mixing bowl
  - Spoon or spatula for mixing
- Airtight jar or container for storage

Method:

Prepare Your Workspace:

- Ensure your workspace is clean and dry. Gather all the necessary ingredients and tools.

Combine Sugar and Oil:

- In a mixing bowl, add the granulated sugar.

- Gradually pour the melted coconut oil over the sugar while stirring continuously. Mix until the sugar is evenly coated with the oil.

Add Essential Oils and Vanilla Extract:

- Add the essential oils and vanilla extract (if using) to the sugar and oil mixture. Stir well to distribute the fragrance evenly.

Check Consistency:

- Check the consistency of the body scrub. It should have a slightly wet and crumbly texture that holds together when pressed.

Transfer to Container:

- Carefully transfer the body scrub into an airtight jar or container for storage. Ensure the container is clean and dry before adding the scrub.

Label and Store:

- Label the jar with the date and type of body scrub. Store it in a cool, dry place away from direct sunlight.

Additional Tips:

- Customization: You can customize your body scrub by adding other ingredients like coffee grounds, oatmeal, or essential oils based on your preferences and skin needs.
- Usage: Use the body scrub in the shower or bath by taking a small amount and gently massaging it onto damp skin in circular motions. Rinse thoroughly with warm water.

This homemade body scrub is excellent for exfoliating and smoothing the skin, leaving it feeling soft and rejuvenated. Adjust the ingredients and scents according to your preferences for a personalized experience.

Ingredients:

- Brown Sugar - 1/2 cup
- Olive Oil - 2 tablespoons (or any carrier oil like almond, jojoba, or coconut oil)
- Honey - 1 tablespoon (optional, for its antibacterial properties)
- Essential Oils - 5-10 drops (such as tea tree oil, lavender, or chamomile)

Equipment/Tools:

- Mixing bowl
- Spoon or spatula for mixing
- Airtight jar or container for storage

Method:

Prepare Your Workspace:

- Ensure your workspace is clean and dry. Gather all the ingredients and tools needed.

Combine Brown Sugar and Oil:

- In a mixing bowl, add the brown sugar.

- Gradually pour the olive oil (or your chosen carrier oil) over the sugar while stirring continuously. Mix until the sugar is coated evenly with the oil.

Add Honey and Essential Oils:

- If using honey, add it to the sugar and oil mixture and stir well to incorporate.

- Add the essential oils of your choice for fragrance and skin benefits. Mix thoroughly.

Check Consistency:

- Check the consistency of the facial scrub. It should have a slightly damp texture that holds together but isn't too oily.

Transfer to Container:

- Carefully transfer the facial scrub into an airtight jar or container for storage. Ensure the container is clean and dry before adding the scrub.

Label and Store:

- Label the jar with the date and type of facial scrub. Store it in a cool, dry place away from direct sunlight.

Additional Tips:

- Skin Sensitivity: Test the facial scrub on a small area of your skin to ensure it doesn't cause any irritation before applying it to your face.
- Usage: Use the facial scrub on damp skin by taking a small amount and gently massaging it onto your face in circular motions. Rinse thoroughly with warm water.

This homemade facial scrub is gentle and exfoliating, helping to remove dead skin cells and leave your face feeling smooth and refreshed. Adjust the ingredients and essential oils based on your skin's needs and sensitivities.

Ingredients:

Carrier Oil (Choose one or a blend) -

- Sweet Almond Oil - 1/4 cup
- Jojoba Oil - 1/4 cup
- Coconut Oil - 1/4 cup (melted)

Essential Oils (Choose one or a blend) -

- Lavender Essential Oil - 10 drops
- Peppermint Essential Oil - 5 drops
- Eucalyptus Essential Oil - 5 drops

Equipment/Tools:

- Dark-colored glass bottle or container with a tight-fitting lid for storage
  - Mixing bowl or measuring cup
- Funnel (optional)

Method:

Prepare Your Workspace:

- Ensure your workspace is clean and dry. Gather all the ingredients and tools needed.

Choose Carrier Oils:

- In a mixing bowl or measuring cup, combine the chosen carrier oils. You can use a single carrier oil or create a blend by mixing different oils.

Add Essential Oils:

- Once you've blended the carrier oils, add the essential oils according to your preference or the desired scent profile. Use a combination of essential oils for fragrance and potential therapeutic benefits.

Mix Thoroughly:

- Stir or gently swirl the oils to ensure they are well combined. If you're using a bottle with a small opening, you might want to use a funnel to pour the mixture into the container.

Transfer to Storage Container:

- Carefully pour the mixed massage oil into a dark-colored glass bottle or container with a tight-fitting lid. Dark-colored glass helps protect the oils from light exposure, which can degrade them over time.

Label and Store:

- Label the bottle with the date and type of massage oil. Store it in a cool, dry place away from direct sunlight.

Additional Tips:

- Testing: Before using the massage oil extensively, perform a patch test on a small area of skin to ensure there are no adverse reactions.
- Usage: Massage oils can be used for body massage or as a moisturizer after a shower or bath. Warm a small amount between your palms before applying it to the skin.

This homemade massage oil offers a wonderful way to unwind and relax, providing the benefits of both the carrier oils and the chosen essential oils. Customize the blend according to your preferences and desired aromatherapy effects.

Ingredients:

Jojoba Oil - 1/2 ounce (or about 1 tablespoon)
Argan Oil - 1/2 ounce (or about 1 tablespoon)
Sweet Almond Oil - 1/2 ounce (or about 1 tablespoon)
Essential Oils (Optional for fragrance and additional benefits):

- Cedarwood Essential Oil - 3 drops
- Sandalwood Essential Oil - 2 drops
- Peppermint Essential Oil - 1 drop

Equipment/Tools:

- Dark-colored glass bottle with a dropper or airtight container for storage
- Mixing bowl or measuring cup
- Funnel (optional)

Method:

Prepare Your Workspace:

- Ensure your workspace is clean and dry. Gather all the ingredients and tools needed.

Combine Carrier Oils:

- In a mixing bowl or measuring cup, carefully measure out the jojoba oil, argan oil, and sweet almond oil. These carrier oils provide nourishment and conditioning to the beard.

Add Essential Oils (Optional):

- If using essential oils for fragrance or additional benefits, add the drops of cedarwood, sandalwood, and peppermint essential oils to the carrier oil mixture. Essential oils should be added sparingly and can be adjusted to suit personal preference.

Mix Thoroughly:

- Stir the oils together gently or use a funnel to pour the mixture into a dark-colored glass bottle or airtight container. Dark-colored glass helps protect the oils from light exposure, preserving their quality.

Label and Store:

- Label the bottle or container with the date and type of beard oil. Store it in a cool, dry place away from direct sunlight.

Additional Tips:

- Patch Test: Before applying the beard oil extensively, perform a patch test on a small area of skin to ensure there are no allergic reactions or irritations.

- Usage: Use the dropper to dispense a few drops of the beard oil onto your palms, rub them together, and then massage the oil into your beard and the skin beneath it. This helps moisturize and condition both the hair and the skin.

This homemade beard oil is a great way to maintain a healthy and well-groomed beard. The carrier oils provide nourishment, while the optional essential oils add fragrance and potential additional benefits for both the beard and the skin. Adjust the blend according to personal preference and skin sensitivity.

Hand Sanitizer

Ingredients:

- Isopropyl Alcohol (Rubbing Alcohol) - 2/3 cup (99% alcohol content)
- Aloe Vera Gel - 1/3 cup (to moisturize and soothe skin)
- Tea Tree Essential Oil - 10 drops (or other essential oils for added antibacterial properties and fragrance)
- Small Squeeze Bottle or Pump Bottle

Equipment/Tools:

- Mixing bowl or measuring cup
- Spoon or whisk for mixing
- Funnel (optional)
- Small squeeze bottle or pump bottle for storage

Method:

Prepare Your Workspace:

- Ensure your workspace is clean and dry. Gather all the ingredients and tools needed.

Measure Isopropyl Alcohol:

- Pour the isopropyl alcohol into a mixing bowl or measuring cup. Ensure it has at least 99% alcohol content for effective sanitization.

Add Aloe Vera Gel:

- Add the aloe vera gel to the alcohol. This helps to moisturize and soothe the skin, counteracting the drying effects of alcohol.

Mix Thoroughly:

- Use a spoon or whisk to thoroughly mix the alcohol and aloe vera gel until they are well combined.

Add Essential Oil:

- Add 10 drops of tea tree essential oil (or another antibacterial essential oil of your choice) to the mixture. Stir again to ensure it's evenly distributed.

Transfer to Storage Container:

- Use a funnel if necessary to carefully pour the hand sanitizer mixture into a small squeeze bottle or pump bottle for easy dispensing.

Label and Store:

- Label the bottle with the contents and date of preparation. Store it in a cool, dry place away from direct sunlight.

Additional Tips:

- Consistency: If the sanitizer is too thick, you can add a little more alcohol to thin it out. If it's too runny, add a bit more aloe vera gel.
- Usage: Apply a small amount of the homemade hand sanitizer to your hands and rub them together until dry. Reapply as needed.

Remember, while homemade hand sanitizers can be effective, it's essential to use them properly and follow the recommended guidelines for hand hygiene from health authorities. This recipe provides a DIY option when commercial sanitizers may not be readily available, but it's important to prioritize thorough handwashing with soap and water whenever possible.

Ingredients:

- Epsom Salt - 2 cups
- Sea Salt or Himalayan Pink Salt - 1/2 cup
- Baking Soda - 1/2 cup
- Essential Oils - 10-15 drops (for fragrance)
- Dried Herbs or Flower Petals - Optional, for added aromatics and visual appeal

Equipment/Tools:

- Mixing bowl
- Spoon or whisk
- Airtight container for storage

Method:

Prepare the Base:

- In a mixing bowl, combine the Epsom salt, sea salt or Himalayan pink salt, and baking soda. Mix them together thoroughly using a spoon or whisk.

Add Essential Oils:

- Add 10-15 drops of your chosen essential oils to the salt mixture. Stir well to evenly distribute the oils throughout the salts. You can adjust the amount of oil depending on your preference for scent strength.

Optional: Add Dried Herbs or Flower Petals:

- If desired, add dried herbs like lavender, chamomile, rosemary, or flower petals to the mixture. These can enhance the aroma and visual appeal of the bath salts. Mix them in well.

Store in an Airtight Container:

- Once the ingredients are thoroughly mixed, transfer the bath salt mixture into an airtight container for storage. Make sure to seal it tightly to preserve the fragrance.

Usage Tips:

- Bath Preparation: Add a handful (about 1/2 cup) of the bath salts to warm bathwater while the tub is filling. Allow the salts to dissolve completely before soaking in the bath.
- Relaxation: The combination of salts and essential oils can help promote relaxation and soothe tired muscles.

Bath salts are a wonderful addition to a relaxing bath routine. Customize the scents by using different essential oil blends or dried herbs according to your preferences. Store the bath salts in a dry place away from moisture to maintain their quality.

Ingredients:

- Witch Hazel - 1/2 cup
  - Aloe Vera Gel - 1/4 cup
- Vegetable Glycerin - 1 tablespoon
- Essential Oils - Optional, for fragrance (e.g., lavender, sandalwood, cedarwood)

Equipment/Tools:

- Mixing bowl or container
  - Whisk or spoon
- Airtight bottle or container for storage

Method:

Combine Ingredients:

- In a mixing bowl or container, combine the witch hazel, aloe vera gel, and vegetable glycerin. Stir the mixture thoroughly using a whisk or spoon until all the ingredients are well incorporated.

Optional: Add Essential Oils:

- If you prefer a scented aftershave, add a few drops of your chosen essential oils to the mixture. Stir well to ensure the oils are evenly distributed.

Transfer to Storage Container:

- Once the ingredients are well mixed, pour the aftershave lotion into an airtight bottle or container suitable for storage.

Usage:

- After shaving, apply a small amount of the aftershave lotion to your skin. Gently massage it into the shaved areas to soothe and hydrate the skin.

Usage Tips:

- Skin Soothing: Witch hazel helps soothe skin irritation, while aloe vera provides hydration and healing properties.
- Fragrance: Essential oils not only add fragrance but also offer additional benefits to the skin.

This homemade aftershave lotion provides a natural and soothing option for post-shave care. Adjust the amount of essential oils based on your preference for fragrance strength. Store the aftershave lotion in a cool, dry place for longevity.

Ingredients for Stick Deodorant:

- Coconut Oil - 3 tablespoons
  - Shea Butter - 2 tablespoons
- Beeswax - 2 tablespoons
- Baking Soda - 3 tablespoons
- Arrowroot Powder or Cornstarch - 3 tablespoons
- Essential Oils - 15-20 drops (for fragrance, optional)

Ingredients for Cream Deodorant:

- Coconut Oil - 1/4 cup
  - Shea Butter - 2 tablespoons
- Arrowroot Powder or Cornstarch - 1/4 cup
- Baking Soda - 2 tablespoons
- Essential Oils - 15-20 drops (for fragrance, optional)

Equipment/Tools:

- Double boiler or makeshift one (a pot and heat-resistant container)
  - Mixing bowl
- Spoon or spatula
- Deodorant container (for stick) or jar (for cream)

Method:

Melt Ingredients:

- Use a double boiler (or a pot with a heat-resistant container inside) to melt the coconut oil, shea butter, and beeswax together over low heat.

Add Dry Ingredients:

- Once melted, remove the mixture from heat. Add the baking soda and arrowroot powder (or cornstarch) to the melted oils. Mix well until a smooth consistency is achieved.

Add Essential Oils:

- If using essential oils for fragrance, add them to the mixture. Stir thoroughly to evenly distribute the oils.

Pour into Container:

- For stick deodorant: Pour the mixture into a deodorant container while it's still liquid. Allow it to cool and solidify.

- For cream deodorant: Pour the mixture into a clean jar or container suitable for storage. It will solidify as it cools.

Usage:

- For stick deodorant: Apply as you would with a commercial stick deodorant, swiping it onto clean, dry underarms.

- For cream deodorant: Use a small amount and apply it to clean, dry underarms with your fingers.

Usage Tips:

- Test Patch: Always perform a patch test on a small area of your skin to ensure you don't have any adverse reactions to the ingredients.
- Consistency: If you prefer a softer or firmer deodorant, adjust the amounts of ingredients accordingly in future batches.

Homemade deodorants provide a natural alternative to commercial products. Adjust the amount of baking soda if you have sensitive skin, as some individuals may be sensitive to it. Store the deodorant in a cool, dry place for use.

Ingredients:

- Fractionated Coconut Oil - 2 tablespoons
  - Witch Hazel - 2 tablespoons
- Filtered Water - 2 tablespoons
- Jojoba Oil - 1 tablespoon (optional, for added moisturizing properties)
- Essential Oils (optional, for fragrance and additional benefits)

Equipment/Tools:

- Mixing bowl or container
  - Stirring utensil
- Airtight bottle or container for storage

Method:

Combine Ingredients:

- In a mixing bowl or container, combine the fractionated coconut oil, witch hazel, filtered water, and jojoba oil (if using). Mix them together thoroughly using a spoon or stirrer.

Optional: Add Essential Oils:

- If desired, add a few drops of essential oils like lavender, chamomile, or tea tree oil for fragrance and additional benefits. Stir well to incorporate them into the mixture.

Transfer to Storage Container:

- Once the ingredients are well mixed, pour the makeup remover solution into an airtight bottle or container suitable for storage.

Usage:

- To use, shake the bottle before each use to ensure the ingredients are well blended. Apply a small amount of the makeup remover to a cotton pad or cloth and gently wipe away makeup from the face.

Usage Tips:

- Gentle Application: Be gentle while using the makeup remover to avoid irritation to the eyes or skin.
- Avoid Contact with Eyes: Ensure the solution doesn't get into the eyes while removing makeup.

This homemade makeup remover is gentle on the skin and effectively removes makeup. It's also customizable based on your preferences for oils and scents. Store it in a cool, dry place and shake well before each use.

Ingredients:

- Acetone - 2/3 cup
- Filtered Water - 1/3 cup
- Glycerin - 1 teaspoon (optional, for moisturizing)

Equipment/Tools:

- Mixing bowl or container
- Stirring utensil
- Airtight bottle or container for storage

Method:

Combine Ingredients:

- In a mixing bowl or container, mix the acetone and filtered water together. Stir well to ensure they are thoroughly combined.

Optional: Add Glycerin:

- If you prefer a nail polish remover with added moisturizing properties, add a teaspoon of glycerin to the acetone-water mixture. Stir to incorporate it evenly.

Transfer to Storage Container:

- Pour the homemade nail polish remover solution into an airtight bottle or container suitable for storage.

Usage:

- To use, soak a cotton ball or pad with the homemade nail polish remover and gently press it onto your nail. Hold it in place for a few seconds to allow the remover to dissolve the nail polish, then wipe the nail in one direction to remove the polish.

Usage Tips:

- Ventilation: Use this nail polish remover in a well-ventilated area due to the acetone's strong odor.
- Moisturizing: Glycerin can help counteract the drying effects of acetone, but if you have sensitive or dry nails, consider applying a moisturizer or cuticle oil after using the remover.

Always ensure that the container used for storage is airtight to prevent evaporation of the acetone. Store the homemade nail polish remover away from heat or flames, as acetone is flammable.

Ingredients:

- Shea Butter - 1/4 cup
  - Coconut Oil - 1/4 cup
- Sweet Almond Oil - 2 tablespoons
- Beeswax Pellets - 2 tablespoons
- Essential Oils - Optional, for fragrance and added benefits (e.g., lavender, chamomile)

Equipment/Tools:

- Double boiler or makeshift one (a pot and heat-resistant container)
  - Mixing bowl
- Hand mixer or whisk
- Airtight container for storage

Method:

Melt Ingredients:

- Use a double boiler or a pot with a heat-resistant container to melt the shea butter, coconut oil, sweet almond oil, and beeswax together over low heat. Stir occasionally until fully melted and combined.

Cool Slightly:

- Remove the mixture from heat and let it cool for a few minutes, but not to the point of solidifying.

Add Essential Oils (Optional):

- If using essential oils for fragrance or additional benefits, add a few drops to the slightly cooled mixture. Stir well to incorporate.

Whip the Cream:

- Transfer the mixture to a mixing bowl. Using a hand mixer or whisk, whip the mixture until it becomes creamy and begins to cool and thicken. This step helps create a lighter, whipped texture for the cream.

Transfer to Container:

- Once whipped to your desired consistency, transfer the hand cream to an airtight container suitable for storage.

Usage:

- Apply the hand cream as needed to moisturize and hydrate your hands.

Usage Tips:

- Storage: Store the hand cream in a cool, dry place away from direct sunlight. Use clean fingers or a scoop/spatula to avoid introducing bacteria into the cream.
- Variations: Experiment with different essential oil blends to create various scents and add specific properties to your hand cream.

This homemade hand cream provides natural hydration and moisturization for dry hands. Customize it by adjusting the amount of essential oils or trying different oils for varied skin benefits. Enjoy the nourishing effects of this DIY hand cream!

Ingredients:

- Coconut Oil - 2 tablespoons
- Honey - 1 tablespoon
- Avocado - 1 ripe avocado
- Egg - 1
- Essential Oil (optional) - A few drops for fragrance and added benefits (e.g., lavender, rosemary)

Equipment/Tools:

- Mixing bowl
- Fork or blender
- Shower cap or plastic wrap
- Towel

Method:

Prepare the Ingredients:

- Mash the ripe avocado in a mixing bowl until it becomes a smooth paste. Add the coconut oil, honey, and egg to the mashed avocado. Mix everything together thoroughly.

Optional: Add Essential Oil:

- If using essential oil for fragrance or added benefits, add a few drops to the mixture and blend well.

Apply the Hair Mask:

- Dampen your hair slightly. Section your hair and apply the mask generously, starting from the roots to the ends. Ensure even coverage.

Cover and Wait:

- Once the hair is coated with the mask, cover it with a shower cap or wrap it with plastic wrap to retain heat and moisture. Leave the mask on for about 20-30 minutes to allow the nutrients to penetrate your hair.

Rinse and Shampoo:

- After the designated time, rinse the hair mask out thoroughly with lukewarm water. Follow up with your regular shampoo and conditioner routine to remove any residue.

Usage Tips:

- Adjust Consistency: If the mask is too thick, add a bit of water or more oil to make it easier to apply.
- Hair Type Consideration: This mask is generally suitable for most hair types, but individuals with oily hair may want to avoid applying the mask to the scalp or use less oil.

This DIY hair mask combines the nourishing properties of avocado, coconut oil, honey, and egg to help moisturize and revitalize your hair. Use it once a week or as needed for an extra boost of hydration and nutrients.

Ingredients:

- Arrowroot Powder or Cornstarch - 2 tablespoons
  - Cocoa Powder or Cinnamon - 1-2 teaspoons (for darker hair, optional)
  - Essential Oil - Optional, for fragrance (e.g., lavender, peppermint)

Equipment/Tools:

- Mixing bowl
  - Spoon or whisk
- Container with a shaker lid or an old clean salt/pepper shaker

Method:

Mix Dry Ingredients:

- In a mixing bowl, combine the arrowroot powder or cornstarch with the cocoa powder or cinnamon (if using). Mix well until evenly blended.

Optional: Add Essential Oil:

- If desired, add a few drops of essential oil to the dry mixture for fragrance. Stir to incorporate the oil evenly.

Transfer to Shaker Container:

- Once thoroughly mixed, transfer the dry shampoo mixture into a container with a shaker lid or an old clean salt/pepper shaker for easy application.

Usage Tips:

● Application: Sprinkle a small amount of the dry shampoo onto the roots of your hair or areas where it appears greasy or oily. Use your fingers to massage the powder into your scalp and hair.

● Blending (for darker hair): If you have darker hair, ensure that the cocoa powder or cinnamon is well blended to avoid visible white residue. You can adjust the amount based on your hair color.

This DIY dry shampoo helps absorb excess oil from your hair, giving it a refreshed look between washes. It's a convenient and quick solution for days when washing your hair isn't an option. Adjust the ingredients to suit your hair color and preference for scent.

Creating homemade sunscreen requires careful consideration of efficacy and safety. However, here's a basic recipe using natural ingredients. Please note that this recipe might not provide the same level of protection as commercial sunscreens:

Ingredients:

- Coconut Oil - 1/4 cup
  - Shea Butter - 1/4 cup
- Jojoba Oil - 1/8 cup
- Zinc Oxide Powder - 2 tablespoons (non-nano, uncoated, and at least 20% zinc oxide)
- Vitamin E Oil - 1 teaspoon
- Essential Oils (optional) - For fragrance and added benefits (e.g., lavender, chamomile)

Equipment/Tools:

- Double boiler or makeshift one (a pot and heat-resistant container)
  - Mixing utensil
- Airtight container for storage

Method:

Melt Oils:

- Use a double boiler or a pot with a heat-resistant container to melt the coconut oil, shea butter, and jojoba oil together over low heat. Stir occasionally until fully melted.

Add Zinc Oxide:

- Once the oils are melted, let the mixture cool slightly. Add the zinc oxide powder slowly, stirring continuously until fully incorporated. Be cautious not to inhale the zinc oxide powder.

Optional: Add Vitamin E and Essential Oils:

- After the mixture has cooled a bit more, add the vitamin E oil and any essential oils for fragrance and added benefits. Stir well to combine.

Transfer to Container:

- Pour the homemade sunscreen mixture into an airtight container suitable for storage.

Usage Tips:

- Stir Before Use: Before using, make sure to stir or shake the sunscreen thoroughly as the zinc oxide might settle at the bottom.
- Patch Test: Always perform a patch test to ensure no allergic reactions occur, especially if using essential oils.
- Reapplication: Reapply the homemade sunscreen frequently, especially after swimming or sweating, as it may not have the same longevity as commercial sunscreens.

Homemade sunscreens might not offer the same level of protection or be as water-resistant as commercially available options. It's essential to use caution and consider alternatives to ensure adequate sun protection, especially during prolonged sun exposure.

Ingredients:

- Witch Hazel - 2 ounces
- Distilled Water - 2 ounces
- Vegetable Glycerin - 1/2 teaspoon
- Essential Oils - Total of 50-60 drops (e.g., citronella, lavender, eucalyptus, peppermint, tea tree)

Equipment/Tools:

- Spray bottle (4-ounce capacity)
- Mixing utensil

Method:

Prepare the Base:

- In a small bowl or mixing container, combine the witch hazel, distilled water, and vegetable glycerin. Mix them together thoroughly.

Add Essential Oils:

- Add 50-60 total drops of essential oils to the base mixture. You can blend different oils according to your preference, ensuring the total drops add up to around 50-60. Stir well to combine.

Transfer to Spray Bottle:

- Using a funnel, pour the bug repellent mixture into a 4-ounce spray bottle.

Usage Tips:

- Shake Well Before Use: Shake the bottle well before each use to ensure the oils are evenly distributed.
- Application: Spray the bug repellent on exposed skin or clothing before heading outdoors. Avoid spraying near eyes or mouth.

This homemade bug repellent offers a natural alternative to commercial insect repellents. Essential oils like citronella, lavender, eucalyptus, peppermint, and tea tree are known for their insect-repelling properties. However, reapplication may be needed more frequently compared to conventional bug repellents. Always perform a patch test to ensure no adverse reactions to the oils.

Ingredients:

- Coconut Oil - 1 tablespoon
- Honey - 1 tablespoon
- Brown Sugar - 2 tablespoons
- Optional: Flavoring - A few drops of vanilla extract or essential oil (e.g., peppermint, lavender) for taste and fragrance

Equipment/Tools:

- Mixing bowl
- Spoon or spatula
- Airtight container for storage

Method:

Combine Ingredients:

- In a mixing bowl, blend the coconut oil, honey, and brown sugar together. Mix until all the ingredients are thoroughly combined.

Optional: Add Flavoring:

- If you'd like to enhance the flavor or scent, add a few drops of vanilla extract or your chosen essential oil to the mixture. Stir well to incorporate.

Transfer to Container:

- Once mixed, transfer the lip scrub into an airtight container suitable for storage.

Usage Tips:

● Application: To use the lip scrub, take a small amount and gently massage it onto your lips using your fingertips. Rub it in a circular motion to exfoliate and remove dry or flaky skin.

● Rinse and Moisturize: After scrubbing for about a minute, rinse your lips with lukewarm water and follow up with a moisturizing lip balm.

This homemade lip scrub helps exfoliate and nourish your lips, leaving them feeling soft and smooth. It's an easy and natural way to maintain smooth lips, especially during dry or cold weather. Store it in a cool, dry place and use it as needed for exfoliation.

Ingredients:

- Distilled Water - 1/2 cup
  - Witch Hazel - 1 tablespoon
- Vegetable Glycerin - 1 teaspoon
- Aloe Vera Gel - 1-2 tablespoons
- Essential Oils (optional) - A few drops for fragrance and additional benefits (e.g., lavender, rose, tea tree)

Equipment/Tools:

- Spray bottle (4-ounce capacity)
  - Mixing bowl or measuring cup
- Stirring utensil

Method:

Prepare the Base:

- In a mixing bowl or measuring cup, combine the distilled water, witch hazel, vegetable glycerin, and aloe vera gel. Stir well to ensure they are thoroughly mixed.

Optional: Add Essential Oils:

- If desired, add a few drops of essential oils for fragrance or added benefits. Stir the mixture again to incorporate the oils evenly.

Transfer to Spray Bottle:

- Using a funnel, pour the homemade setting spray mixture into a 4-ounce spray bottle.

Usage Tips:

● Shake Before Use: Shake the bottle well before each use to ensure all the ingredients are mixed properly.

● Application: After applying makeup, hold the bottle about 6-8 inches away from your face and spray lightly. Allow it to air dry without touching your face.

This DIY makeup setting spray can help set your makeup, providing a more long-lasting and fresh look. The ingredients are gentle and can offer some additional benefits to your skin. Remember to store the spray bottle in a cool, dry place and use it as part of your makeup routine as needed.

Ingredients:

- Flaxseeds - 1/4 cup
- Water - 2 cups
- Essential Oils (optional) - A few drops for fragrance (e.g., lavender, rosemary)

Equipment/Tools:

- Medium saucepan
- Stirring utensil
- Fine-mesh strainer or cheesecloth
- Airtight container for storage

Method:

Boil the Flaxseeds:

- In a medium saucepan, combine the flaxseeds and water. Bring the mixture to a boil over medium heat, stirring occasionally.

Simmer and Stir:

- Once boiling, reduce the heat to low and let the mixture simmer for about 10-15 minutes. Stir occasionally to prevent the seeds from sticking to the bottom of the pan.

Strain the Gel:

- Remove the saucepan from heat and let the mixture cool slightly. Strain the gel through a fine-mesh strainer or cheesecloth into a bowl to separate the seeds from the gel. Squeeze the strainer or cloth to extract as much gel as possible.

Optional: Add Essential Oils:

- If desired, add a few drops of essential oils to the strained gel for fragrance. Stir well to incorporate.

Transfer to Container:

- Pour the homemade hair gel into an airtight container suitable for storage.

Usage Tips:

- Application: Use a small amount of the gel and apply it to damp or dry hair to style as desired.
- Storage: Store the hair gel in the refrigerator. Due to the natural ingredients, it may have a shorter shelf life compared to commercial gels.

This DIY hair gel made from flaxseeds offers a natural alternative for styling hair. It provides hold without the harsh chemicals found in some commercial hair products. Experiment with the amount used to achieve your desired hold and style.

Ingredients:

- Fractionated Coconut Oil - 2 tablespoons
- Argan Oil - 1 tablespoon
- Jojoba Oil - 1 tablespoon
- Vitamin E Oil - 1 teaspoon
- Essential Oils (optional) - A few drops for fragrance and added benefits (e.g., lavender, rosemary)

Equipment/Tools:

- Mixing bowl or container
- Stirring utensil
- Airtight bottle or container for storage

Method:

Combine Oils:

- In a mixing bowl or container, blend the fractionated coconut oil, argan oil, jojoba oil, and vitamin E oil together. Stir well to ensure all oils are thoroughly mixed.

Optional: Add Essential Oils:

- If using essential oils for fragrance or added benefits, add a few drops to the oil mixture. Stir well to incorporate the oils evenly.

Transfer to Container:

- Once mixed, pour the homemade hair serum into an airtight bottle or container suitable for storage.

Usage Tips:

● Application: Use a small amount of the serum and apply it to damp or dry hair, focusing on the ends or areas prone to dryness. Avoid applying too much to prevent weighing down the hair.

● Storage: Store the hair serum in a cool, dry place away from direct sunlight. Shake well before each use to ensure all the oils are properly mixed.

This DIY hair serum is designed to nourish and moisturize the hair, giving it a healthy and shiny appearance. The combination of oils can help tame frizz and protect hair from damage. Adjust the quantity of essential oils to suit your preference for scent and enjoy the natural benefits of this homemade hair serum.

Beard Balm

Ingredients:

- Shea Butter - 2 tablespoons
  - Beeswax - 2 tablespoons (grated or in pellet form)
- Jojoba Oil - 1 tablespoon
- Coconut Oil - 1 tablespoon
- Essential Oils - A few drops for fragrance (e.g., cedarwood, sandalwood, tea tree)

Equipment/Tools:

- Double boiler or makeshift one (a pot and heat-resistant container)
  - Mixing utensil
- Airtight container for storage

Method:

Melt Ingredients:

- Use a double boiler or a pot with a heat-resistant container to melt the shea butter, beeswax, jojoba oil, and coconut oil together over low heat. Stir occasionally until fully melted and combined.

Optional: Add Essential Oils:

- Once melted, remove the mixture from heat and let it cool slightly. Add a few drops of essential oils for fragrance. Stir well to distribute the oils evenly.

Pour into Container:

- Carefully pour the melted mixture into an airtight container suitable for storage. Allow it to cool and solidify.

Usage Tips:

● Application: Scrape a small amount of the beard balm using your thumbnail. Rub it between your palms to melt it slightly, then massage it into your beard and skin. Style as desired.

● Storage: Store the beard balm in a cool, dry place away from direct sunlight.

This homemade beard balm helps condition, tame, and style facial hair while nourishing the skin underneath. The natural ingredients provide moisture and control for a well-groomed beard. Experiment with different essential oil combinations for various scents and benefits.

Ingredients:

- Liquid Castile Soap: ½ cup
  - Sweet Almond Oil: 2 tablespoons
- Jojoba Oil: 1 tablespoon
- Essential Oil (optional, for fragrance): 10-15 drops (e.g., cedarwood, sandalwood, lavender)
- Distilled Water: ½ cup
- Honey (optional, for added moisture): 1 teaspoon

Tools and Equipment:

- Mixing bowl
  - Whisk or spoon
- Measuring cups/spoons
- Pump bottle or squeeze bottle for storage

Method:

- Prepare Your Workspace: Clean and sanitize your workspace and tools to ensure proper hygiene.
- Measure Ingredients: Measure out the liquid castile soap, sweet almond oil, jojoba oil, and optional honey into a mixing bowl.
- Mix Oils and Soap: Use a whisk or spoon to thoroughly mix the oils and soap together. Ensure that the oils are well incorporated into the soap base.
- Add Essential Oils (Optional): If using essential oils for fragrance, add them to the mixture. Stir well to distribute the fragrance evenly.
- Add Distilled Water: Slowly pour the distilled water into the mixture while stirring continuously. This helps to dilute the soap and oils properly.
- Final Mixing: Whisk or stir the mixture until all the ingredients are well blended. Make sure there are no clumps or separation.

- Transfer to Container: Using a funnel, carefully pour the prepared beard wash into a clean pump bottle or squeeze bottle for storage. Ensure the container is airtight to preserve the product.

- Label and Store: Label the container with the date of preparation and any necessary usage instructions. Store the beard wash in a cool, dry place away from direct sunlight.

Tips:

- Adjust Consistency: If you prefer a thicker or thinner consistency, you can adjust the amount of water used.

- Patch Test: Before regular use, perform a patch test on a small area of skin to ensure no allergic reactions occur.

- Shake Before Use: Some separation may occur between uses, so shake the bottle well before using the beard wash.

This recipe offers a basic beard wash that can be easily prepared at home and scaled up for small-scale production. Remember to adhere to safety guidelines, use quality ingredients, and consider packaging and labeling for a professional touch if planning to sell these products.

Ingredients:

- Jojoba Oil: 1 tablespoon
  - Sweet Almond Oil: 1 tablespoon
  - Vitamin E Oil (optional, for added nourishment): ½ teaspoon
  - Lavender Essential Oil (optional, for fragrance): 4-5 drops
  - Rosemary Essential Oil (optional, for strengthening): 3-4 drops

Tools and Equipment:

- Mixing bowl
  - Measuring spoons
  - Dropper bottle or small, clean glass container with a tight lid for storage

Method:

- Prepare Your Workspace: Ensure your workspace and tools are clean and sanitized for making the cuticle oil.
- Measure Ingredients: Measure out the jojoba oil and sweet almond oil into a mixing bowl. If you're using vitamin E oil and essential oils, measure those as well.
- Mix Oils: Combine the jojoba oil and sweet almond oil in the mixing bowl. If using, add the vitamin E oil at this stage. Mix the oils thoroughly.
- Add Essential Oils (Optional): If you desire a scented cuticle oil or wish to incorporate specific essential oils for nail health, add them to the oil mixture. Stir gently to combine.
- Transfer to Storage Container: Using a small funnel or a steady hand, carefully pour the prepared cuticle oil into a dropper bottle or a clean glass container with a tight lid.
- Label and Store: Label the container with the date of preparation and any necessary usage instructions. Store the cuticle oil in a cool, dark place to maintain its potency.

Tips:

- Customization: Feel free to adjust the essential oil quantities according to your preference for fragrance or nail health benefits.
- Shake Before Use: Before using the cuticle oil, give the bottle a gentle shake to ensure the oils are well mixed.
- Application: Apply a small amount to each nail and massage it into the cuticles. It's best used before bedtime to allow the oil to absorb overnight.

This homemade cuticle oil provides natural nourishment and moisture to keep your cuticles healthy and hydrated. It's a simple product that can be made in small batches for personal use or potentially for sale in a small-scale production setup. Always ensure that your ingredients are of good quality and properly stored for longevity.

Ingredients:

- Carrier Oil (such as Sweet Almond Oil, Jojoba Oil, or Grapeseed Oil): ½ cup
- Essential Oils (for fragrance and therapeutic benefits): 15-20 drops total (e.g., lavender, eucalyptus, chamomile)

Tools and Equipment:

- Mixing bowl
  - Measuring cup/spoons
- Stirring utensil
- Glass bottle or container for storage

Method:

- Prepare Your Workspace: Ensure your workspace and tools are clean and sanitized for making the bath oils.
- Select Carrier Oil: Choose your preferred carrier oil (e.g., sweet almond oil) as the base for your bath oil. Measure out ½ cup of the carrier oil and pour it into a mixing bowl.
- Add Essential Oils: Select your desired essential oils for fragrance and therapeutic benefits. Add 15-20 drops of essential oils to the carrier oil. You can mix different oils for a customized scent or therapeutic effect.
- Mix Thoroughly: Use a stirring utensil to gently mix the carrier oil and essential oils. Ensure that the essential oils are evenly distributed throughout the carrier oil.
- Transfer to Storage Container: Using a funnel or a steady hand, carefully pour the prepared bath oil into a clean glass bottle or container suitable for storage.
- Label and Store: Label the container with the date of preparation and the types of essential oils used. Store the bath oil in a cool, dry place away from direct sunlight.

Tips:

- Skin Sensitivity: Perform a patch test before using the bath oil, especially if you have sensitive skin or allergies to certain essential oils.

- Usage: Add a few drops of the bath oil to your bathwater for a fragrant and moisturizing bathing experience. You can also use it as a massage oil after your bath.

- Variations: Experiment with different combinations of essential oils to create unique scents or to target specific purposes like relaxation or revitalization.

This homemade bath oil is a simple yet luxurious addition to a self-care routine. It can be easily produced in small batches at home and scaled up for small-scale production with minimal equipment and space requirements. Always ensure you're using high-quality oils and properly store the product for longevity and efficacy.

Ingredients:

- Liquid Castile Soap: ½ cup
  - Vegetable Glycerin: ¼ cup
  - Essential Oil (optional, for fragrance): 10-15 drops (e.g., lavender, chamomile, citrus)

Tools and Equipment:

- Mixing bowl
  - Measuring cups/spoons
- Whisk or spoon
- Airtight container for storage

Method:

- Prepare Your Workspace: Ensure your workspace and tools are clean and sanitized for making the bubble bath.
- Measure Ingredients: Measure out the liquid castile soap and vegetable glycerin into a mixing bowl.
- Mix Ingredients: Combine the liquid castile soap and vegetable glycerin in the mixing bowl. Use a whisk or spoon to gently mix the ingredients together. Ensure they are thoroughly blended.
- Add Essential Oil (Optional): If you desire a scented bubble bath, add 10-15 drops of your chosen essential oil into the mixture. Stir well to distribute the fragrance evenly.
- Transfer to Storage Container: Using a funnel or a steady hand, carefully pour the prepared bubble bath mixture into an airtight container suitable for storage.
- Label and Store: Label the container with the date of preparation and any necessary usage instructions. Store the bubble bath in a cool, dry place away from direct sunlight.

Tips:

● Bubble Production: Test the bubble bath by pouring a small amount under running water. Adjust the ingredients if you want more or fewer bubbles.

● Skin Sensitivity: Perform a patch test before using the bubble bath, especially if you have sensitive skin or allergies to certain essential oils.

● Shake Before Use: Some separation may occur between uses, so shake the container gently before each use to remix the ingredients.

This homemade bubble bath offers a delightful and natural way to enjoy a relaxing bath while avoiding harsh chemicals often found in commercial products. It can be produced in small quantities at home and potentially scaled up for small-scale production. Ensure you're using high-quality ingredients and proper storage to maintain the product's quality over time.

Ingredients:

- Liquid Castile Soap: 1 cup
  - Vegetable Glycerin: ½ cup
- Aloe Vera Gel: ¼ cup
- Essential Oil (for fragrance, optional): 15-20 drops (e.g., lavender, peppermint, citrus)

Tools and Equipment:

- Mixing bowl
  - Measuring cups/spoons
- Whisk or spoon
- Airtight container for storage

Method:

- Prepare Your Workspace: Ensure your workspace and tools are clean and sanitized for making the shower gel.
- Measure Ingredients: Measure out the liquid castile soap, vegetable glycerin, and aloe vera gel into a mixing bowl.
- Combine Ingredients: Add the liquid castile soap, vegetable glycerin, and aloe vera gel into the mixing bowl. Use a whisk or spoon to gently blend the ingredients together. Mix until they are thoroughly combined.
- Add Essential Oil (Optional): If you want scented shower gel, add 15-20 drops of your chosen essential oil into the mixture. Stir well to distribute the fragrance evenly.
- Test and Adjust: Test the consistency and scent of the shower gel. If needed, you can add more soap for a thicker consistency or more essential oil for a stronger scent.
- Transfer to Storage Container: Using a funnel or a steady hand, carefully pour the prepared shower gel into an airtight container suitable for storage.

● Label and Store: Label the container with the date of preparation and any necessary usage instructions. Store the shower gel in a cool, dry place away from direct sunlight.

Tips:

● Shake Before Use: Some separation may occur between uses, so shake the container gently before each use to mix the ingredients.

● Customization: Feel free to experiment with different essential oils or adjust the ratios of ingredients to suit your preferences.

● Patch Test: Before regular use, perform a patch test on a small area of skin to ensure no allergic reactions occur.

This homemade shower gel provides a natural and gentle cleansing experience without harsh chemicals. It's suitable for personal use and can potentially be produced in small batches for a small-scale production setup. Always use quality ingredients and proper storage to maintain the shower gel's quality over time.

Ingredients:

- Witch Hazel: ½ cup
  - Rose Water: ½ cup
- Aloe Vera Gel: 2 tablespoons
- Essential Oil (optional, for additional benefits or fragrance): 5-10 drops (e.g., tea tree, lavender)

Tools and Equipment:

- Mixing bowl
  - Measuring cup/spoons
- Whisk or spoon
- Spray bottle or airtight container for storage

Method:

- Prepare Your Workspace: Ensure your workspace and tools are clean and sanitized for making the face toner.
- Measure Ingredients: Measure out the witch hazel, rose water, and aloe vera gel into a mixing bowl.
- Combine Ingredients: Add the witch hazel, rose water, and aloe vera gel into the mixing bowl. Use a whisk or spoon to gently mix the ingredients together. Stir until they are thoroughly combined.
- Add Essential Oil (Optional): If you wish to incorporate essential oils for added benefits or fragrance, add 5-10 drops of your chosen essential oil into the mixture. Stir well to distribute the oil evenly.
- Transfer to Storage Container: Using a funnel or a steady hand, carefully pour the prepared face toner into a spray bottle or airtight container suitable for storage.
- Label and Store: Label the container with the date of preparation and any necessary usage instructions. Store the face toner in a cool, dry place away from direct sunlight.

Tips:

● Shake Before Use: Before each use, shake the bottle gently to ensure the ingredients are well mixed.

● Application: Apply the toner to a cotton pad and gently swipe it over your face after cleansing. It helps to remove excess oil, dirt, and balance the skin's pH.

● Skin Sensitivity: Perform a patch test before using the face toner, especially if you have sensitive skin or allergies to certain ingredients.

This homemade face toner is a gentle and natural way to refresh and tone your skin. It can be easily produced in small quantities at home and potentially scaled up for small-scale production. Always ensure the ingredients used are of good quality and properly stored to maintain the toner's efficacy over time.

Ingredients:

- Jojoba Oil: 1 tablespoon
- Rosehip Seed Oil: 1 tablespoon
- Argan Oil: 1 tablespoon
- Vitamin E Oil: ½ teaspoon
- Essential Oils (optional, for added benefits): 5-10 drops (e.g., frankincense, lavender, tea tree)

Tools and Equipment:

- Mixing bowl
- Measuring spoons
- Dropper bottle or glass container with a tight lid for storage

Method:

- Prepare Your Workspace: Ensure your workspace and tools are clean and sanitized for making the face serum.
- Measure Ingredients: Measure out the jojoba oil, rosehip seed oil, argan oil, and vitamin E oil into a mixing bowl.
- Combine Ingredients: Add all the measured oils into the mixing bowl. Gently stir or whisk the oils together to ensure they are thoroughly blended.
- Add Essential Oils (Optional): If using essential oils for added benefits or fragrance, add 5-10 drops of your chosen essential oil into the oil mixture. Stir well to distribute the essential oils evenly.
- Transfer to Storage Container: Using a funnel or a steady hand, carefully pour the prepared face serum into a dropper bottle or a clean glass container with a tight lid for storage.
- Label and Store: Label the container with the date of preparation and any necessary usage instructions. Store the face serum in a cool, dry place away from direct sunlight.

Tips:

- Shake Before Use: Before using the face serum, give the bottle a gentle shake to ensure all the oils are well mixed.

- Application: Apply a few drops of the serum onto clean skin and gently massage it in. It can be used in the morning or evening as part of your skincare routine.

- Patch Test: Perform a patch test on a small area of skin before using the face serum regularly, especially if you have sensitive skin or allergies to certain ingredients.

This homemade face serum is a nourishing blend of oils that can offer hydration and various skin benefits. It's suitable for personal use and can potentially be produced in small batches for a small-scale production setup. Always use high-quality oils and store the serum properly to maintain its efficacy over time.

Ingredients:

- Liquid Castile Soap: ¼ cup
  - Raw Honey: 1 tablespoon
- Jojoba Oil: 1 tablespoon
- Filtered Water: ¼ cup
- Essential Oil (optional, for fragrance): 5-10 drops (e.g., tea tree, lavender, chamomile)

Tools and Equipment:

- Mixing bowl
  - Measuring cups/spoons
- Whisk or spoon
- Pump bottle or airtight container for storage

Method:

- Prepare Your Workspace: Ensure your workspace and tools are clean and sanitized for making the face cleanser.
- Measure Ingredients: Measure out the liquid castile soap, raw honey, jojoba oil, filtered water, and optional essential oil into a mixing bowl.
- Combine Ingredients: Add the liquid castile soap, raw honey, jojoba oil, and filtered water into the mixing bowl. Use a whisk or spoon to gently mix the ingredients together. Stir until they are thoroughly combined.
- Add Essential Oil (Optional): If desired, add 5-10 drops of your chosen essential oil into the mixture. Stir well to distribute the fragrance evenly.
- Test and Adjust: Test the consistency and scent of the face cleanser. If needed, you can adjust the ratios of ingredients to suit your preferences.
- Transfer to Storage Container: Using a funnel or a steady hand, carefully pour the prepared face cleanser into a pump bottle or airtight container suitable for storage.

• Label and Store: Label the container with the date of preparation and any necessary usage instructions. Store the face cleanser in a cool, dry place away from direct sunlight.

Tips:

● Shake Before Use: Before each use, gently shake the container to ensure the ingredients are well mixed.

• Application: Pump a small amount of the cleanser onto your palm, lather with water, and gently massage it onto your face. Rinse thoroughly with water.

• Skin Sensitivity: Perform a patch test before using the face cleanser, especially if you have sensitive skin or allergies to certain ingredients.

This homemade face cleanser is gentle and natural, suitable for various skin types. It can be produced in small quantities at home and potentially scaled up for small-scale production. Always use high-quality ingredients and store the cleanser properly to maintain its effectiveness over time.

Ingredients:

- Coconut Oil: 1 tablespoon
- Sweet Almond Oil: 1 tablespoon
- Shea Butter: 1 tablespoon
- Beeswax: ½ tablespoon
- Vitamin E Oil: ½ teaspoon
- Essential Oil (optional, for additional benefits): 3-5 drops (e.g., rosehip, chamomile, frankincense)

Tools and Equipment:

- Double boiler or heat-safe bowl and saucepan
- Mixing spoon
- Small jars or containers for storage

Method:

- Prepare Your Workspace: Ensure your workspace and tools are clean and sanitized for making the eye cream.
- Melt Solid Ingredients: Use a double boiler or a heat-safe bowl placed over a saucepan with simmering water. Add the coconut oil, sweet almond oil, shea butter, and beeswax to the bowl. Allow the ingredients to melt gently, stirring occasionally with a mixing spoon.
- Incorporate Vitamin E Oil: Once the mixture is fully melted and combined, remove it from heat. Add the vitamin E oil to the melted mixture and stir well to incorporate.
- Add Essential Oil (Optional): If desired, add 3-5 drops of your chosen essential oil into the mixture. Stir well to distribute the oil evenly.
- Allow Cooling: Let the mixture cool for a few minutes. It should start to thicken as it cools.

• Transfer to Containers: Carefully pour or spoon the prepared eye cream into small jars or containers suitable for storage. Ensure the containers are clean and airtight.

• Label and Store: Label the containers with the date of preparation and any necessary usage instructions. Store the eye cream in a cool, dry place away from direct sunlight.

Tips:

• Patch Test: Before applying the eye cream near the eyes, perform a patch test on a small area of skin to check for any adverse reactions.

• Application: Apply a small amount of the eye cream onto your ring finger and gently dab it around the eye area, avoiding direct contact with the eyes.

• Storage: Keep the eye cream sealed properly and use it within a few months for best results.

This homemade eye cream is nourishing and gentle, suitable for the delicate skin around the eyes. It can be produced in small quantities at home and potentially scaled up for small-scale production. Always use high-quality ingredients and proper storage to maintain the cream's effectiveness over time.

Ingredients:

- Shea Butter: 2 tablespoons
- Coconut Oil: 1 tablespoon
- Jojoba Oil: 1 tablespoon
- Aloe Vera Gel: 1 tablespoon
- Vitamin E Oil: ½ teaspoon
- Essential Oil (optional, for fragrance): 5-10 drops (e.g., lavender, geranium, rose)

Tools and Equipment:

- Double boiler or heat-safe bowl and saucepan
- Mixing spoon or whisk
- Small jars or containers for storage

Method:

- Prepare Your Workspace: Ensure your workspace and tools are clean and sanitized for making the face moisturizer.
- Melt Solid Ingredients: Use a double boiler or a heat-safe bowl placed over a saucepan with simmering water. Add the shea butter and coconut oil to the bowl. Allow them to melt gently, stirring occasionally with a mixing spoon or whisk.
- Incorporate Liquid Ingredients: Once the shea butter and coconut oil are melted, remove the mixture from heat. Add the jojoba oil, aloe vera gel, and vitamin E oil. Stir well to combine all the ingredients thoroughly.
- Add Essential Oil (Optional): If desired, add 5-10 drops of your chosen essential oil into the mixture. Stir well to distribute the oil evenly.
- Allow Cooling: Let the mixture cool down for a few minutes. It will start to solidify as it cools.

• Transfer to Containers: Carefully pour or spoon the prepared face moisturizer into small jars or containers suitable for storage. Ensure the containers are clean and airtight.

• Label and Store: Label the containers with the date of preparation and any necessary usage instructions. Store the face moisturizer in a cool, dry place away from direct sunlight.

Tips:

• Patch Test: Before using the face moisturizer on your face, perform a patch test on a small area of skin to check for any allergic reactions.

• Application: Use a small amount of the moisturizer and gently massage it into your skin. It's best to apply it after cleansing your face.

• Storage: Keep the moisturizer sealed properly and use it within a few months for optimal freshness.

This homemade face moisturizer is nourishing and can be adjusted to suit different skin types. It's suitable for personal use and can potentially be produced in small batches for a small-scale production setup. Always use high-quality ingredients and store the moisturizer properly to maintain its effectiveness over time.

Ingredients:

- Aloe Vera Gel: 1 tablespoon
- Witch Hazel: 1 tablespoon
- Glycerin: ½ teaspoon
- Silicone-Free Face Lotion: 1 teaspoon
- Cornstarch or Arrowroot Powder: ½ teaspoon
- Foundation or BB Cream (optional, for tint): ½ teaspoon
- Vitamin E Oil (optional, for added benefits): 2-3 drops

Tools and Equipment:

- Mixing bowl
- Measuring spoons
- Whisk or spoon
- Small container for storage

Method:

- Prepare Your Workspace: Ensure your workspace and tools are clean and sanitized for making the makeup primer.
- Combine Ingredients: In a mixing bowl, add the aloe vera gel, witch hazel, glycerin, silicone-free face lotion, and cornstarch or arrowroot powder.
- Mix Thoroughly: Use a whisk or spoon to blend all the ingredients together. Stir until the mixture is smooth and well combined.
- Optional: Add Foundation or BB Cream: If you prefer a tinted primer, add ½ teaspoon of foundation or BB cream into the mixture. Blend it thoroughly to achieve an even color.
- Add Vitamin E Oil (Optional): If desired, add a few drops of vitamin E oil for added skincare benefits. Stir to incorporate it evenly into the mixture.

- Transfer to Storage Container: Carefully pour or spoon the prepared makeup primer into a small container suitable for storage. Ensure the container is clean and airtight.

- Label and Store: Label the container with the date of preparation and any necessary usage instructions. Store the makeup primer in a cool, dry place away from direct sunlight.

Tips:

- Application: Apply a small amount of the primer onto clean, moisturized skin before makeup application. Allow it to set for a minute or two before applying foundation.

- Skin Sensitivity: Perform a patch test before using the primer, especially if you have sensitive skin or allergies to certain ingredients.

- Customization: Adjust the consistency by adding more aloe vera gel for a thinner primer or more powder for a thicker consistency.

This homemade makeup primer provides a smooth base for makeup application and can be tailored to suit individual preferences. It's suitable for personal use and can potentially be produced in small quantities for personal use or as part of a small-scale production setup. Always use high-quality ingredients and proper storage to maintain the primer's effectiveness over time.

Makeup Foundation

Ingredients:

- Zinc Oxide (Non-nano): 1 tablespoon
- Arrowroot Powder: 1 tablespoon
- Cocoa Powder or Cinnamon (for shade/tint): Adjust as needed for desired color
- Bentonite Clay or Kaolin Clay: ½ teaspoon
- Jojoba Oil: ½ teaspoon
- Shea Butter: ½ teaspoon
- Essential Oil (optional, for fragrance): 2-3 drops (e.g., lavender, chamomile)

Tools and Equipment:

- Mixing bowl
- Measuring spoons
- Mortar and pestle or grinder (for powder blending)
- Small container or compact for storage

Method:

- Prepare Your Workspace: Ensure your workspace and tools are clean and sanitized for making the makeup foundation.
- Mix Dry Ingredients: In a mixing bowl, combine the zinc oxide, arrowroot powder, cocoa powder or cinnamon (for shade), and bentonite or kaolin clay. Use a mortar and pestle or grinder to blend the dry ingredients thoroughly and achieve a smooth consistency.
- Melt Shea Butter: In a separate heat-safe bowl, melt the shea butter using a double boiler or a microwave in short bursts. Once melted, set it aside to cool slightly.
- Incorporate Oils: Add the jojoba oil to the melted shea butter and stir to combine.

- Combine Dry and Liquid Ingredients: Slowly pour the liquid mixture into the bowl with the dry ingredients. Mix thoroughly using a spoon or spatula until a smooth, creamy texture is achieved.

- Adjust Consistency and Color: If needed, add more arrowroot powder for a thicker consistency or more cocoa powder/cinnamon for a darker shade. Mix well until the desired consistency and color are reached.

- Add Essential Oil (Optional): If desired, add a few drops of your chosen essential oil for fragrance. Stir to incorporate evenly into the foundation mixture.

- Transfer to Storage Container: Carefully spoon or pour the prepared makeup foundation into a small container or a compact suitable for storage. Ensure the container is clean and airtight.

- Label and Store: Label the container with the date of preparation and any necessary usage instructions. Store the makeup foundation in a cool, dry place away from direct sunlight.

Tips:

- Application: Apply the foundation using a makeup brush, sponge, or your fingertips, blending it evenly onto your skin.

- Skin Sensitivity: Perform a patch test before using the foundation, especially if you have sensitive skin or allergies to certain ingredients.

- Shelf Life: Use the foundation within a few months for optimal freshness.

This homemade makeup foundation offers a customizable and natural alternative to commercial foundations. It can be produced in small quantities for personal use or potentially as part of a small-scale production setup. Always use high-quality ingredients and proper storage to maintain the foundation's effectiveness over time. Adjust the recipe according to your skin tone and preferences for coverage and consistency.

Ingredients:

- Arrowroot Powder or Cornstarch: 1 tablespoon
  - Beetroot Powder (for blush) or Cocoa Powder (for bronzer): Adjust quantity for desired shade
  - Cinnamon (for bronzer, optional): Adjust quantity for desired shade
  - Nutmeg (for bronzer, optional): Adjust quantity for desired shade
  - Jojoba Oil or Almond Oil: ½ teaspoon
  - Essential Oil (optional, for fragrance): 2-3 drops (e.g., rose, lavender)

Tools and Equipment:

- Mixing bowl
  - Measuring spoons
  - Mortar and pestle or grinder (for powder blending)
  - Small container or compact for storage

Method:

- Prepare Your Workspace: Ensure your workspace and tools are clean and sanitized for making the blush/bronzer.
- Mix Dry Ingredients: In a mixing bowl, combine the arrowroot powder or cornstarch with the primary pigment powder (beetroot powder for blush or cocoa powder for bronzer). Use a mortar and pestle or grinder to blend the dry ingredients thoroughly, achieving a smooth consistency.
- Adjust Shade (for Bronzer): If making bronzer, add cinnamon and nutmeg to the mixture gradually until you achieve the desired shade. Blend well to ensure an even distribution of color.
- Incorporate Oils: Add the jojoba oil or almond oil to the dry mixture. Stir or mix well until the oil is evenly distributed and the mixture has a smooth texture.
- Optional: Add Essential Oil: If desired, add a few drops of your chosen essential oil for fragrance. Stir to incorporate evenly into the mixture.

- Check and Adjust Consistency: Test the consistency by pressing a small amount of the mixture between your fingers. If it's too dry, add a little more oil. If too wet, add a touch more powder.
- Transfer to Storage Container: Carefully spoon or pour the prepared blush/bronzer into a small container or a compact suitable for storage. Ensure the container is clean and airtight.
- Label and Store: Label the container with the date of preparation and any necessary usage instructions. Store the blush/bronzer in a cool, dry place away from direct sunlight.

Tips:

- Application: Use a makeup brush to apply the blush or bronzer to your cheeks or desired areas for a natural-looking glow.
- Skin Sensitivity: Perform a patch test before using the blush/bronzer, especially if you have sensitive skin or allergies to certain ingredients.
- Customization: Adjust the pigment ratios to achieve your desired shade and intensity.

This homemade blush/bronzer offers a natural alternative to commercial makeup products. It can be produced in small quantities for personal use or potentially as part of a small-scale production setup. Always use high-quality ingredients and proper storage to maintain the blush/bronzer's effectiveness over time. Adjust the recipe according to your desired color and consistency preferences.

Ingredients:

- Arrowroot Powder or Cornstarch: 1 tablespoon
- Mica Powder (various colors for desired shades): Adjust quantity for desired shade and color
- Jojoba Oil or Almond Oil: ½ teaspoon
- Witch Hazel or Rubbing Alcohol (optional): Few drops (for pressed eyeshadow)

Tools and Equipment:

- Mixing bowl
- Measuring spoons
- Small jars or containers for loose eyeshadow OR empty eyeshadow pans for pressed eyeshadow
- Spoon or spatula for mixing
- Small dropper (if using witch hazel or rubbing alcohol for pressed eyeshadow)

Method for Loose Eyeshadow:

- Prepare Your Workspace: Ensure your workspace and tools are clean and sanitized for making the eyeshadow.
- Mix Dry Ingredients: In a mixing bowl, combine the arrowroot powder or cornstarch with the mica powder(s) of your choice. Use a spoon or spatula to blend the dry ingredients thoroughly, achieving the desired shade.
- Incorporate Oils: Add the jojoba oil or almond oil to the dry mixture. Mix well until the oil is evenly distributed and the mixture has a smooth, consistent texture.
- Check Consistency: Test the consistency by pressing a small amount of the mixture between your fingers. It should hold together without being too crumbly or too wet. Adjust by adding more powder or oil as needed.

- Transfer to Storage Containers: Carefully spoon or pour the prepared eyeshadow into small jars or containers suitable for loose eyeshadow. Ensure the containers are clean and airtight.

Method for Pressed Eyeshadow (Optional):

Follow steps 1-4 above to prepare the eyeshadow mixture.
- Add a few drops of witch hazel or rubbing alcohol into the mixture, using a dropper. Mix until the consistency resembles wet sand.
- Transfer the wet eyeshadow mixture into empty eyeshadow pans or compacts, pressing it firmly into the pans using a clean spoon or spatula.
- Let the pressed eyeshadow dry and set for a few hours or overnight before using it.

Tips:

Application: Use an eyeshadow brush to apply the loose eyeshadow or pressed eyeshadow to your eyelids.
- Skin Sensitivity: Perform a patch test before using the eyeshadow, especially if you have sensitive skin or allergies to certain ingredients.
- Customization: Experiment with different mica powder shades to create your desired eyeshadow colors.

This homemade eyeshadow provides a natural alternative to commercial makeup products. It can be produced in small quantities for personal use or potentially as part of a small-scale production setup. Always use high-quality ingredients and proper storage to maintain the eyeshadow's effectiveness over time. Adjust the recipe according to your desired color and consistency preferences.

Ingredients:

- Activated Charcoal (for black mascara): ½ teaspoon
- Bentonite Clay: ¼ teaspoon
- Coconut Oil: ½ teaspoon
- Beeswax: ½ teaspoon
- Aloe Vera Gel: ½ teaspoon
- Vitamin E Oil: 2-3 drops

Tools and Equipment:

- Double boiler or heat-safe bowl and saucepan
- Small container or mascara tube (clean and sterilized)
- Small spatula or spoon for mixing
- Small brush or mascara wand

Method:

- Prepare Your Workspace: Ensure your workspace and tools are clean and sanitized for making the mascara.
- Melt Ingredients: Use a double boiler or a heat-safe bowl placed over a saucepan with simmering water. Add the coconut oil and beeswax to the bowl. Allow them to melt gently, stirring occasionally with a small spatula or spoon.
- Add Aloe Vera and Vitamin E: Once melted, remove the mixture from heat. Add the aloe vera gel and vitamin E oil to the melted ingredients. Stir well to combine all the ingredients thoroughly.
- Incorporate Charcoal and Clay: Gradually add the activated charcoal and bentonite clay into the mixture, stirring continuously. Mix until you achieve a smooth, consistent texture.
- Transfer to Container: Carefully pour or spoon the prepared mascara mixture into a clean and sterilized container or mascara tube suitable for storage. Ensure the container is airtight.

• Cool and Set: Let the mascara cool and set for a few hours or overnight before use. This will allow it to thicken and achieve the proper consistency.

• Use a Mascara Wand: Once the mascara has set, use a clean mascara wand or brush to apply it to your eyelashes.

Tips:

• Application: Apply the homemade mascara as you would any other mascara, starting at the base of your lashes and wiggling the wand upward.

• Skin Sensitivity: Perform a patch test before using the mascara, especially if you have sensitive skin or allergies to certain ingredients.

• Shelf Life: Use the mascara within a few months for optimal freshness.

This homemade mascara offers a natural alternative to commercial products. It can be produced in small quantities for personal use or potentially as part of a small-scale production setup. Always use high-quality ingredients and proper storage to maintain the mascara's effectiveness over time. Adjust the recipe according to your desired consistency and color preferences.

Ingredients:

- Activated Charcoal (for black eyeliner): ½ teaspoon
- Coconut Oil: ½ teaspoon
- Shea Butter: ½ teaspoon
- Beeswax: ½ teaspoon
- Aloe Vera Gel: ½ teaspoon
- Vitamin E Oil: 2-3 drops

Tools and Equipment:

- Double boiler or heat-safe bowl and saucepan
- Small container or eyeliner pot (clean and sterilized)
- Small spatula or spoon for mixing
- Eyeliner brush or angled brush

Method:

- Prepare Your Workspace: Ensure your workspace and tools are clean and sanitized for making the eyeliner.
- Melt Ingredients: Use a double boiler or a heat-safe bowl placed over a saucepan with simmering water. Add the coconut oil, shea butter, and beeswax to the bowl. Allow them to melt gently, stirring occasionally with a small spatula or spoon.
- Add Aloe Vera and Vitamin E: Once melted, remove the mixture from heat. Add the aloe vera gel and vitamin E oil to the melted ingredients. Stir well to combine all the ingredients thoroughly.
- Incorporate Activated Charcoal: Gradually add the activated charcoal into the mixture, stirring continuously. Mix until you achieve a smooth, consistent texture.
- Transfer to Container: Carefully pour or spoon the prepared eyeliner mixture into a clean and sterilized container or eyeliner pot suitable for storage. Ensure the container is airtight.

● Cool and Set: Let the eyeliner cool and set for a few hours or overnight before use. This will allow it to thicken and achieve the proper consistency for application.

● Use an Eyeliner Brush: Once the eyeliner has set, use a clean eyeliner brush or angled brush to apply it to your eyelids.

Tips:

● Application: Apply the homemade eyeliner as you would any other eyeliner, starting from the inner corner of your eye and drawing along your lash line.

● Skin Sensitivity: Perform a patch test before using the eyeliner, especially if you have sensitive skin or allergies to certain ingredients.

● Shelf Life: Use the eyeliner within a few months for optimal freshness.

This homemade eyeliner provides a natural alternative to commercial products. It can be produced in small quantities for personal use or potentially as part of a small-scale production setup. Always use high-quality ingredients and proper storage to maintain the eyeliner's effectiveness over time. Adjust the recipe according to your desired consistency and color preferences.

Ingredients for Lipstick:

- Beeswax: 1 tablespoon
  - Shea Butter: 1 tablespoon
- Coconut Oil: 1 tablespoon
- Cocoa Powder or Beetroot Powder (for color): Adjust quantity for desired shade
- Essential Oil (optional, for fragrance): 2-3 drops (e.g., peppermint, vanilla)

Ingredients for Lip Gloss:

- Coconut Oil: 1 tablespoon
  - Beeswax: 1 tablespoon
- Sweet Almond Oil: 1 tablespoon
- Mica Powder or Food-Grade Cosmetic Pigment (for color): Adjust quantity for desired shade
- Flavoring Oil (optional, for flavor): 2-3 drops (e.g., cherry, strawberry)

Tools and Equipment:

- Double boiler or heat-safe bowl and saucepan
  - Small containers or lip balm tubes for lipsticks/lip gloss (clean and sterilized)
- Small spatula or spoon for mixing
- Dropper (for lip gloss)

Method for Lipstick:

- Prepare Your Workspace: Ensure your workspace and tools are clean and sanitized for making the lipstick.
- Melt Ingredients: Use a double boiler or a heat-safe bowl placed over a saucepan with simmering water. Add the beeswax, shea butter, and coconut

oil to the bowl. Allow them to melt gently, stirring occasionally with a small spatula or spoon.

- Incorporate Color: Once melted, remove the mixture from heat. Add the cocoa powder or beetroot powder gradually, mixing well until you achieve the desired shade.

- Add Fragrance (Optional): If desired, add a few drops of your chosen essential oil for fragrance. Stir to incorporate evenly into the mixture.

- Transfer to Containers: Carefully pour or spoon the prepared lipstick mixture into clean and sterilized containers or lip balm tubes suitable for storage. Ensure the containers are airtight.

Method for Lip Gloss:

- Follow steps 1-3 above to melt the beeswax, coconut oil, and sweet almond oil.

- Incorporate the mica powder or cosmetic pigment into the melted mixture, stirring continuously until you achieve the desired color.

- Add flavoring oil (if desired) to the mixture and stir well.

- Use a dropper to transfer the lip gloss mixture into clean and sterilized containers suitable for storage. Ensure the containers are airtight.

Tips:

- Application: Use a lip brush or your fingertip to apply the homemade lipstick or lip gloss to your lips.

- Skin Sensitivity: Perform a patch test before using the lipstick/lip gloss, especially if you have sensitive skin or allergies to certain ingredients.

- Shelf Life: Use the lipstick or lip gloss within a few months for optimal freshness.

These homemade lipstick and lip gloss recipes offer natural alternatives to commercial products. They can be produced in small quantities for personal use or potentially as part of a small-scale production setup. Always use high-quality ingredients and proper storage to maintain the effectiveness and freshness of the lipstick or lip gloss over time. Adjust the recipe according to your desired color, consistency, and fragrance preferences.

Ingredients:

- Shea Butter: ½ cup
  - Cocoa Butter: ¼ cup
- Coconut Oil: ¼ cup
- Sweet Almond Oil or Jojoba Oil: 2 tablespoons
- Essential Oil (optional, for fragrance): 15-20 drops (e.g., lavender, citrus)

Tools and Equipment:

- Double boiler or heat-safe bowl and saucepan
  - Hand mixer or stand mixer
- Mixing bowl
- Clean and sterilized jars or containers for storage

Method:

- Prepare Your Workspace: Ensure your workspace and tools are clean and sanitized for making the body butter.
- Melt Solid Ingredients: Use a double boiler or a heat-safe bowl placed over a saucepan with simmering water. Add the shea butter, cocoa butter, and coconut oil to the bowl. Allow them to melt gently, stirring occasionally with a spoon or spatula.
- Incorporate Liquid Oil: Once the solid ingredients are melted, remove the mixture from heat. Add the sweet almond oil or jojoba oil into the mixture. Stir well to combine all the ingredients thoroughly.
- Cool Down: Let the mixture cool for about 20-30 minutes at room temperature. It should start to solidify slightly around the edges but remain soft in the center.
- Add Essential Oil: If desired, add the essential oil drops into the partially cooled mixture. Stir gently to distribute the essential oil evenly.

- Whip the Body Butter: Using a hand mixer or a stand mixer, whip the mixture on medium to high speed for about 5-10 minutes until it becomes fluffy and achieves a creamy texture.

- Transfer to Containers: Carefully spoon or pour the whipped body butter into clean and sterilized jars or containers suitable for storage. Ensure the containers are airtight.

- Label and Store: Label the containers with the date of preparation and any necessary usage instructions. Store the body butter in a cool, dry place away from direct sunlight.

Tips:

- Application: Apply a small amount of the body butter to your skin and massage gently. It's best used after a shower or bath when your skin is slightly damp.

- Skin Sensitivity: Perform a patch test before using the body butter, especially if you have sensitive skin or allergies to certain ingredients.

- Shelf Life: Use the body butter within several months for optimal freshness.

This homemade body butter provides nourishment and moisture to the skin. It can be produced in small quantities for personal use or potentially as part of a small-scale production setup. Always use high-quality ingredients and proper storage to maintain the body butter's effectiveness over time. Adjust the recipe according to your preferences and skin needs.

Baby Shampoo/Body Wash

Ingredients:

- Liquid Castile Soap (unscented): ½ cup
- Distilled Water: ½ cup
- Sweet Almond Oil or Olive Oil: 1 tablespoon
- Vegetable Glycerin: 1 tablespoon
- Essential Oil (optional, for fragrance): 5-10 drops of lavender or chamomile (ensure it's safe for babies)

Tools and Equipment:

- Mixing bowl
- Measuring cup and spoon
- Clean and sterilized container or bottle for storage
- Stirring utensil (spoon or whisk)

Method:

- Prepare Your Workspace: Ensure your workspace and tools are clean and sanitized for making the baby shampoo/body wash.
- Mixing the Ingredients: In a mixing bowl, combine the liquid castile soap, distilled water, sweet almond oil or olive oil, and vegetable glycerin. Gently stir the ingredients together using a spoon or whisk until well combined.
- Optional Fragrance: If using essential oil for fragrance, add 5-10 drops of a baby-safe essential oil such as lavender or chamomile to the mixture. Stir again to distribute the fragrance evenly.
- Transfer to Storage Container: Carefully pour the prepared baby shampoo/body wash into a clean and sterilized container or bottle suitable for storage. Ensure the container has a tight-fitting lid to prevent spillage.
- Label and Store: Label the container with the date of preparation and any necessary usage instructions. Store the baby shampoo/body wash in a cool, dry place.

Tips:

● Application: Use a small amount of the homemade baby shampoo/body wash during bath time. Apply it gently to your baby's hair and body, avoiding contact with the eyes.

● Skin Sensitivity: Perform a patch test before using the baby shampoo/body wash, especially if your baby has sensitive skin or allergies to certain ingredients.

● Shelf Life: Use the baby shampoo/body wash within a few months for optimal freshness.

This homemade baby shampoo/body wash provides a gentle and natural cleansing option for your little one. It can be produced in small quantities for personal use or potentially as part of a small-scale production setup. Always use high-quality ingredients and ensure they are suitable for your baby's delicate skin. Adjust the recipe and fragrance according to your preferences and any sensitivities your baby might have.

Diaper Rash Cream

Ingredients:

- Coconut Oil: ¼ cup
- Shea Butter: 2 tablespoons
- Zinc Oxide Powder: 2 tablespoons
- Beeswax: 1 tablespoon
- Lavender Essential Oil (optional): 10-15 drops (ensure it's safe for babies)

Tools and Equipment:

- Double boiler or heat-safe bowl and saucepan
- Mixing bowl
- Clean and sterilized container for storage
- Stirring utensil (spoon or spatula)

Method:

- Prepare Your Workspace: Ensure your workspace and tools are clean and sanitized for making the diaper rash cream.
- Melt Ingredients: Use a double boiler or a heat-safe bowl placed over a saucepan with simmering water. Add the coconut oil, shea butter, and beeswax to the bowl. Allow them to melt gently, stirring occasionally with a spoon or spatula until fully melted and combined.
- Incorporate Zinc Oxide: Once melted, remove the mixture from heat. Add the zinc oxide powder to the melted mixture. Stir well to ensure it's fully incorporated and no clumps remain.
- Optional Essential Oil: If using lavender essential oil for added soothing properties and fragrance, add 10-15 drops to the mixture. Stir again to distribute the essential oil evenly.
- Transfer to Storage Container: Carefully pour or spoon the prepared diaper rash cream into a clean and sterilized container suitable for storage. Ensure the container has a tight-fitting lid.

- Cool and Set: Let the cream cool and set at room temperature for a few hours or until it solidifies.
- Label and Store: Label the container with the date of preparation and any necessary usage instructions. Store the diaper rash cream in a cool, dry place away from direct sunlight.

Tips:

- Application: Apply a thin layer of the homemade diaper rash cream to clean and dry skin during diaper changes to help soothe and protect against rashes.
- Skin Sensitivity: Perform a patch test before using the diaper rash cream, especially if your baby has sensitive skin or allergies to certain ingredients.
- Shelf Life: Use the cream within a few months for optimal freshness.

This homemade diaper rash cream provides a natural and protective solution for your baby's sensitive skin. It can be produced in small quantities for personal use or potentially as part of a small-scale production setup. Always use high-quality ingredients and ensure they are suitable for your baby's skin. Adjust the recipe according to your preferences and any sensitivities your baby might have.

Ingredients:

- Carrier Oil (options):

  - Grapeseed Oil
  - Sweet Almond Oil
  - Fractionated Coconut Oil
  - Jojoba Oil
  - Olive Oil
  - *Select one*: ½ cup

- Vitamin E Oil (optional, for added skin benefits): 1 teaspoon
- Chamomile Essential Oil (optional, for fragrance and soothing properties): 5-10 drops (ensure it's safe for babies)

Tools and Equipment:

- Mixing bowl
  - Clean and sterilized bottle for storage
- Funnel (optional)
- Stirring utensil (spoon or spatula)

Method:

- Prepare Your Workspace: Ensure your workspace and tools are clean and sanitized for making the baby oil.
- Mixing the Ingredients: In a mixing bowl, pour your selected carrier oil (grapeseed oil, sweet almond oil, fractionated coconut oil, jojoba oil, or olive oil).
- Optional Vitamin E Oil: If using vitamin E oil for added skin benefits, add 1 teaspoon to the carrier oil. Stir gently to combine.

- Optional Chamomile Essential Oil: If using chamomile essential oil for fragrance and soothing properties, add 5-10 drops to the oil mixture. Stir again to distribute the fragrance evenly.

- Transfer to Storage Bottle: Carefully pour the prepared baby oil into a clean and sterilized bottle suitable for storage. A funnel can be used to make the transfer easier. Ensure the bottle has a tight-fitting lid to prevent spillage.

- Label and Store: Label the bottle with the date of preparation and any necessary usage instructions. Store the baby oil in a cool, dry place away from direct sunlight.

Tips:

- Application: Use the homemade baby oil for gentle massages or as a moisturizer for your baby's skin after bath time.

- Skin Sensitivity: Perform a patch test before using the baby oil, especially if your baby has sensitive skin or allergies to certain ingredients.

- Shelf Life: The baby oil can last for several months to a year if properly stored.

This homemade baby oil provides a natural and nourishing option for your baby's delicate skin. It can be produced in small quantities for personal use or potentially as part of a small-scale production setup. Always use high-quality ingredients and ensure they are suitable for your baby's skin. Adjust the recipe according to your preferences and any sensitivities your baby might have.

Ingredients:

- Shea Butter: ½ cup
- Coconut Oil: ¼ cup
- Sweet Almond Oil or Jojoba Oil: 2 tablespoons
- Beeswax: 2 tablespoons
- Vitamin E Oil: 1 teaspoon
- Chamomile Essential Oil (optional, for fragrance and soothing properties): 5-10 drops (ensure it's safe for babies)

Tools and Equipment:

- Double boiler or heat-safe bowl and saucepan
- Mixing bowl
- Clean and sterilized jar or container for storage
- Hand mixer or stand mixer (optional)
- Stirring utensil (spoon or spatula)

Method:

- Prepare Your Workspace: Ensure your workspace and tools are clean and sanitized for making the baby lotion.
- Melt Ingredients: Use a double boiler or a heat-safe bowl placed over a saucepan with simmering water. Add the shea butter, coconut oil, sweet almond oil or jojoba oil, and beeswax to the bowl. Allow them to melt gently, stirring occasionally with a spoon or spatula until fully melted and combined.
- Incorporate Vitamin E Oil: Once melted, remove the mixture from heat. Add the vitamin E oil to the mixture. Stir well to ensure it's fully incorporated.
- Optional Essential Oil: If using chamomile essential oil for fragrance and soothing properties, add 5-10 drops to the mixture. Stir again to distribute the fragrance evenly.
- Cool Down: Let the mixture cool for a few minutes until it starts to thicken but is still pourable.

- Mixing (Optional): If desired, you can use a hand mixer or stand mixer to whip the mixture for a few minutes until it becomes creamy and smooth.
- Transfer to Storage Container: Carefully pour or spoon the prepared baby lotion into a clean and sterilized jar or container suitable for storage. Ensure the container has a tight-fitting lid.
- Label and Store: Label the container with the date of preparation and any necessary usage instructions. Store the baby lotion in a cool, dry place away from direct sunlight.

Tips:

- Application: Use the homemade baby lotion to moisturize your baby's skin after baths or whenever needed.
- Skin Sensitivity: Perform a patch test before using the baby lotion, especially if your baby has sensitive skin or allergies to certain ingredients.
- Shelf Life: The lotion can last for several months if properly stored.

This homemade baby lotion provides a natural and nourishing option for your baby's delicate skin. It can be produced in small quantities for personal use or potentially as part of a small-scale production setup. Always use high-quality ingredients and ensure they are suitable for your baby's skin. Adjust the recipe according to your preferences and any sensitivities your baby might have.

Reusable Makeup Remover Pads

Materials:

- Fabric: Soft, absorbent fabric such as organic cotton, flannel, or bamboo fabric
- Sewing Thread: Matching or contrasting thread
- Sewing Machine or Needle and Thread: For sewing

Tools:

- Scissors
- Sewing pins
- Sewing needle (if sewing by hand)
- Template (optional, for consistent size)

Method:

- Prepare Fabric: Wash and dry the fabric before cutting to preshrink it. This ensures the finished pads won't shrink after their first wash.
- Cutting Fabric: Using scissors and a template if desired, cut the fabric into circles or squares. Aim for sizes that are convenient for removing makeup (typically 3-4 inches in diameter).
- Layering Fabric: For each pad, layer two pieces of fabric together, placing their right sides facing each other. Pin them in place around the edges, leaving a small opening (about 1-2 inches) to turn the pad right side out.
- Sewing: Sew along the pinned edges, leaving the small opening unsewn. Use a backstitch at the beginning and end to secure the seam. If sewing by hand, use a whip stitch or running stitch.
- Trimming and Turning: Trim any excess fabric around the edges, making sure not to cut the stitches. Turn the pads right side out through the opening.
- Closing Opening: Use a hand stitch or machine stitch to close the small opening. Ensure the seam is neatly closed.
- Finishing: Press the pads with an iron if needed to smooth out any wrinkles.

- Storage: Store the finished reusable makeup remover pads in a clean container or pouch.

Tips:

- Experiment with different fabric types to find what works best for your skin and makeup removal needs.
- Make several pads to have a rotation available between washes.
- Wash the pads in a mesh laundry bag or dedicated pouch to keep them together in the washing machine.

These homemade reusable makeup remover pads are gentle on the skin, reduce waste, and can be washed and reused multiple times. Customize the size and shape to your preference and enjoy their eco-friendly benefits!

Ingredients:

- Soap Base: You can use a melt-and-pour soap base or make soap from scratch using lye (caustic soda) and oils (like coconut oil, olive oil, or shea butter). For beginners, a melt-and-pour soap base is easier and safer.
- Botanicals: Dried lavender flowers, calendula petals, or other botanicals of choice
- Essential Oils: Lavender essential oil, calendula essential oil, or other preferred scents (optional)
- Colorants (optional): Natural colorants like turmeric or spirulina powder (for aesthetic appeal)

Tools and Equipment:

- Double boiler or microwave for melting soap base
  - Soap molds
- Mixing utensils (stainless steel or heat-resistant plastic)
- Cutting knife or soap cutter
- Spray bottle with rubbing alcohol (to prevent bubbles)

Method:

- Prepare Botanicals: If using dried lavender flowers or calendula petals, ensure they are finely ground or chopped for even distribution in the soap. Set aside.
- Melt Soap Base: Cut the melt-and-pour soap base into smaller chunks for easier melting. Use a double boiler or microwave in short bursts to melt the soap base gently. Stir occasionally until fully melted and smooth.
- Add Botanicals and Essential Oils: Once melted, add the finely chopped botanicals and essential oils to the soap base. Stir gently to distribute evenly. Add colorants if desired, but keep in mind that botanicals might alter the soap's color.

• Pour into Molds: Carefully pour the soap mixture into soap molds. Lightly spray the surface with rubbing alcohol to eliminate air bubbles.

• Cool and Set: Allow the soap to cool and harden in the molds for several hours or according to the instructions for the specific soap base used.

• Remove from Molds: Once the soap has completely cooled and solidified, gently remove it from the molds. If using a silicone mold, flex it to release the soap. For other molds, tap the sides to loosen the soap.

• Curing (if using cold-process soap): If you're making soap from scratch using lye, it needs to cure for several weeks before use to ensure saponification is complete and the soap is mild.

• Packaging: Once cured or cooled, package your handcrafted botanical soaps in airtight containers or wrap them in parchment paper for storage or gifting.

Safety Precautions:

● When working with lye to make soap from scratch, use protective gear such as gloves and goggles. Follow proper safety procedures for handling lye.

Enjoy the process of creating beautifully scented handcrafted botanical soaps! Adjust the recipe and scents to suit your preferences and explore various botanical combinations for unique soaps.

www.ingramcontent.com/pod-product-compliance
Lightning Source LLC
Chambersburg PA
CBHW052036150726

48002CB00002B/638